# What Researchers are Saying About the Subject of Traumatic Incident Reduction and Related Techniques:

"We are very impressed with the power and simplicity of TIR in helping trauma sufferers work through their frightening experiences and find great relief."

— Charles R. Figley, PhD, editor of *TRAUMATOLOGY*

"Being able to watch someone go from confusion to certainty, from sadness to happiness in a single session is a wonderful privilege. It is invigorating. I get the same satisfaction and joy from teaching Metapsychology techniques to others."

— Lori Beth Bisbey, PhD, Chartered Counselling Psychologist

"TIR does not require years of collegiate study to pre-qualify the provision of assistance to others. The efficacy of TIR is not contingent on the unique talents of a particular facilitator. The procedure is standardized and does not require continuous adjustments."

— Wendy Coughlin, PhD

"In many cases, TIR results in the complete and permanent elimination of PTSD symptomatology. [My] dissertation suggests the use of TIR as an effective technique in the treatment of child and adolescent Post Traumatic Stress Disorder with the identified population."

— Francine Odio, PhD

"…in TIR you do no interpretation for the client. You do not say to your client: 'That's probably related to something that happened in your childhood.' You would not presume to know what happened; you would not in fact interpret those things for the person."

— Joyce Carbonell, PhD., Florida State University

"The comments given by female inmates [in this study] suggest that they were highly appreciative of the client-respectful nature of TIR. For many of them, this was their first experience with a treatment provider who was both effective and respectful."

— Pamela Vest Valentine, PhD

"This process may activate memories of important details of the recent trauma that heretofore have been omitted or forgotten. In this way, TIR makes use of verbally mediated generalization gradients, which will broaden the exposure treatment stimuli and thus reduce the likelihood of renewal."          — Phillip M. Massad PhD and Timothy L. Hulsey, PhD

# Traumatic Incident Reduction:
# Research and Results
## 2nd Edition

## Edited by Victor R. Volkman
### Public Information Chair, TIR Association

First Edition:  April 2005 (ISBN-13 978-1-932690-11-8)

Second Edition: March 2008 (ISBN-13 978-1-932690-50-7)

---

Library of Congress Cataloging-in-Publication Data

Traumatic incident reduction : research and results / edited by Victor R. Volkman. -- 2nd ed.
   p. ; cm. --  (Explorations in metapsychology series)
 Includes bibliographical references and index.
 ISBN-13: 978-1-932690-50-7 (trade paper : alk. paper)
 ISBN-10: 1-932690-50-6 (trade paper : alk. paper)
 1.  Post-traumatic stress disorder. 2.  Stress management. 3.  Crisis intervention (Mental health services)  I. Volkman, Victor R. II. Series: Explorations in metapsychology.
 [DNLM: 1.  Stress Disorders, Post-Traumatic--therapy--Collected Works.  WM 170 T777468 2008]
 RC552.P67T75555 2008
 616.85'21--dc22

                    2007051748

---

Distributed by:
Baker & Taylor, Ingram Book Group, New Leaf Distributing Co.

Published by:
Loving Healing Press
5145 Pontiac Trail
Ann Arbor, MI 48105
USA

http://www.LovingHealing.com or
info@LovingHealing.com
Fax +1 734 663 6861

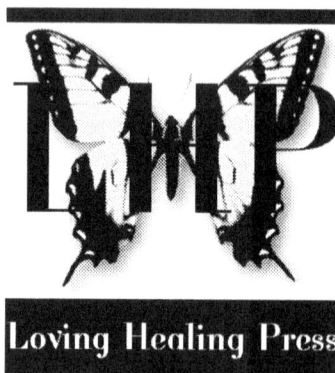

Loving Healing Press

## Explorations in Metapsychology Series:

- *Beyond Trauma: Conversations on Traumatic Incident Reduction, 2nd Edition* by Victor R. Volkman
- *Life Skills: How to Improve the Quality of Your Life with Metapsychology* by Marian K. Volkman
- *Traumatic Incident Reduction: Research & Results, Ed. by Victor R. Volkman*
- *Coping with Crisis: A Counselor's Guide to* Restabilization by Jim Burtles
- *Traumatic Incident Reduction, 2nd Ed* by French & Harris

## TIR Applications Series:

- *Children and Traumatic Incident Reduction: Creative and Cognitive Approaches* by Marian K. Volkman
- *Traumatic Incident Reduction and Critical Incident Stress Management: A Synergistic Approach* by Victor R. Volkman

## Series Editor: Robert Rich, Ph.D.

*"To be what we are,
and to become what we are capable of becoming,
is the only end in life"*

**—Robert Louis Stevenson (June 1880)**

## *About our Series Editor, Robert Rich, Ph.D.*

Loving Healing Press is pleased to announce Robert Rich, Ph.D. as Series Editor for the *Explorations in Metapsychology Series*. This exciting new series plans to bring you the best of Metapsychology in practical application, theory, and self-help formats.

Robert Rich, M.Sc., Ph.D., M.A.P.S., A.A.S.H. is a highly experienced counseling psychologist. His web site www.anxietyanddepression-help.com is a storehouse of helpful information for people suffering from almost any way we can make ourselves and each other unhappy.

Bob is also a multiple award-winning writer of both fiction and non-fiction, and a professional editor. His writing is displayed at www.bobswriting.com. You are advised not to visit him there unless you have the time to get lost for a while.

Two of his books are tools for psychological self-help: *Anger and Anxiety: Be in charge of your emotions and control phobias* and *Personally Speaking: Single session email therapy*. However, his philosophy and psychological knowledge come through in all his writing, which is perhaps why three of his books have won international awards, and he has won many minor prizes. Dr. Rich currently resides in Wombat Hollow in Australia.

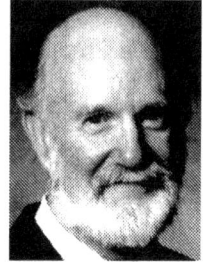

In memory of

**Stephen Bisbey (1952–2004)**

Counselor, trainer, author, and beloved friend of the
many people he worked with and helped.

# Table of Contents

# Introduction: A Brief History of
# TIR Research and Results

The purpose of *Traumatic Incident Reduction: Research & Results* is to summarize the major outcomes of the first decade of research on this subject (approximately 1994 to 2004). TIR as a formal subject came on the scene in 1988 with the publication of *Beyond Psychology: An Introduction to Metapsychology (1ˢᵗ Ed.)* by Frank A. Gerbode, M.D. This book codified a straightforward step-by-step technique for handling the effects of multiple past traumas connected by similarity of incident or theme. Of course, TIR did not spring into existence by itself and is the product of diverse influences and the input of many authors. As Robert H. Moore, Ph.D. points out in his essay "Psychological Foundations of TIR", there are clear antecedents and concepts borrowed from imaginal flooding, desensitization, repetitive review, Rogerian techniques, and Pavlov, just to name a few.

Following the introduction of TIR and workshop-level training in the late 1980s, there came a flood of anecdotal evidence of the efficacy of TIR. Among the most dramatic of the early successes involved Post-Traumatic Stress Disorder (PTSD) in Vietnam combat veterans (see *Beyond Trauma: Conversations on Traumatic Incident Reduction, 2ⁿᵈ Ed,* 2005). Please note that TIR can be applied to the vast majority of traumatic stress cases and is not limited to the particular diagnosis of PTSD. However, a mountain of anecdotes does not a scientific research project make.

In the early 1990s, two researchers began independent studies of TIR as part of their doctoral dissertation work. In the UK, Lori Beth Bisbey began a groundbreaking study of traumatic stress in crime victims and how TIR alleviated their symptoms. This study showed for the first time the advantage of TIR over Direct Therapeutic Exposure techniques. Shortly thereafter, Wendy Coughlin employed TIR facilitators around the United States in a study of how anxiety and panic attack symptoms might be relieved by TIR. Both dissertations were published in 1995 and brief summaries appear in this book.

During this same period (1994), Charles R. Figley and Joyce Carbonell of Florida State University developed the "Active Ingredient" study. The purpose of this research was to analyze four brief treatments for traumatic stress [1] (TIR, V/KD, EMDR, TFT) and hopefully discover or distill the common element which made them effective. Two summaries of this research appear in this book.

Pamela V. Valentine built on the results of Bisbey and Coughlin with her outcome study on a controlled study of incarcerated females in Florida prisons. This study was published as a dissertation in 1997 and is also summarized in this book. In this study, the experimental condition showed a statistically significant decrease in symptoms of posttraumatic stress disorder (and its

---

[1] Traumatic Incident Reduction (TIR), Visual Kinesthetic/Disassociation (V/KD), Eye Movement Desensitization and Reprocessing (EMDR), and Thought Field Therapy (TFT).

related subscales) and of depression and anxiety, while those in the control condition remained approximately the same. Subjects assigned to the experimental condition improved on the measure of self-efficacy at a statistically significant level, while subjects assigned to the control condition did not.

1998-99 saw the publication of the first two textbooks devoted solely to teaching the principles and methods of TIR. In the USA, Gerald French and Chrys Harris published *Traumatic Incident Reduction* as part of the Innovations in Psychology series (CRC Press, Series Editor: Charles R. Figley). In the UK, the team of Stephen and Lori Beth Bisbey published *Brief Therapy for Post-Traumatic Stress Disorder: Traumatic Incident Reduction and Related Techniques* as part of the Brief Therapy and Counselling Series (Wiley, Series Editor: Windy Dryden). As I write this introduction, preparations are underway for the release of a greatly revised second edition of French and Harris' book in late 2005.

Although not a research project, I have included the work of Teresa Descilo, MSW because it is the first published outcome results of TIR with middle-school aged children. Beginning in 2001, this project has shown significant results in reducing post-traumatic and depression symptoms in this vulnerable population of at-risk students.

It is my most fervent hope that in presenting summaries of TIR research data that it will inspire others to back and look at the original studies and consider taking TIR research to the next level of scrutiny and validation. If you would like to learn more about the philosophical roots of TIR or read selected case histories, I highly recommend you peruse *Beyond Trauma: Conversations on Traumatic Incident Reduction, 2nd Ed.* (2005) after reading this book.

**Victor R. Volkman (victor@tir.org)**
**Public Information Chair, TIR Association**
**April 15th, 2005**

# Preface to the 2nd Edition

It has been my great pleasure to collect additional materials for the 2nd Edition of TIR: Research & Results over the past two years. We are proud to present new material in this edition for which we have obtained reprint permissions:

- "A Qualitative Study of Client Perceptions of Traumatic Incident Reduction (TIR): A Brief Trauma Treatment", *Crisis Intervention*, Vol. 4, pp. 1-12 (January 1998) by Pamela Vest Valentine, PhD and Thomas Edward Smith, PhD.

- "Researching PTSD: Going for the Cure" in *Family Therapy Networker* (July-Aug 1996) by Mary Sykes Wylie

- "Exposure Therapy Renewed" Journal of Psychotherapy Integration (2006). Vol. 16, No. 4, 417–428 by Phillip M. Massad and Timothy L. Hulsey

- "Resolving Distress: Exposing A Medical Myth" by John Durkin (2006) from *Proceedings of the 5th Annual Rocky Mountain Region Disaster Mental Health Conference.*

# 1 TIR: Primary Resolution of the Post–Traumatic Stress Disorder

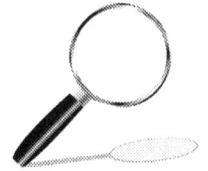

## By Robert H. Moore, Ph.D.

## About the Author

Dr. Moore is a licensed marriage and family therapist, school psychologist and mental health counselor with graduate degrees in counseling psychology from Lehigh (1965) and Walden (1977) Universities. He is a Fellow and Diplomate of the American Board of Medical Psychotherapists; a Diplomate of the International Academy of Behavioral Medicine, Counseling and Psychotherapy.

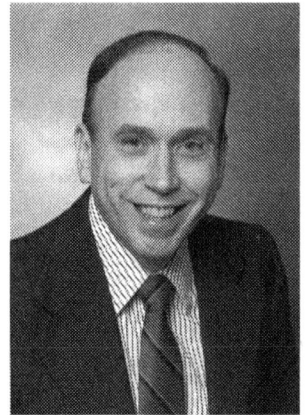

With over thirty years of practice, seventeen as Director of the Institute for Rational Living in Florida, he has co-edited or contributed to six popular books by Albert Ellis; authored chapters on various applications of Cognitive Behavior Therapy and Traumatic Incident Reduction for professional texts by Windy Dryden, Larry Hill and Janet Wolfe; hosted his own nationally syndicated daily talk radio program; and produced over three hundred psychologically-topical news and public service segments for radio and television. He most recently operated a Domestic Violence Intervention Program in Clearwater under contract to Florida's Department of Corrections.

## Problem Profile

In the early 1990's, significant media attention was given to the Post-Traumatic Stress Disorders (PTSD) of Vietnam veterans, whose post-war "nervous" problems (i.e., sleep disturbances, hypervigilance, paranoia, panic attacks explosive rages, and intrusive thoughts) were known to veterans of earlier campaigns as "battle fatigue," "shell shock," and "war neurosis" (Kelly, 1985). As any number of mugging, rape, and accident victims have demonstrated, however, one need not have been a casualty of war to experience the problem (APA, 1987). PTSD appears in children as well as adults (Eth & Pynoos, 1985) and has been attributed to abuse, abortions, burns, broken bones, surgery, rape, overwhelming loss, animal attacks, drug overdoses, near drowning, bullying, intimidation, and similar traumata. It manifests as a wide range of anxieties, insecurities, phobias, panic disorders, anger and rage reactions, guilt complexes, mood and personality anomalies, depressive reactions, self-esteem problems, somatic complaints, and compulsions.

The PTSD reaction is most easily distinguished from emotional problems of other sorts by its signature flashback: the involuntary and often agonizing recall of a past traumatic incident. It can be triggered by an almost limitless variety of present cognitive and perceptual cues (Kilpatrick, 1985; Foa, 1989). Lodged like a startle response beyond conscious control, the reaction frequently catapults its victims into a painful dramatization of an earlier trauma and routinely either distorts or eclipses their perception of present reality. Although we can't confirm that any of the countless animal species with which researchers have replicated Pavlov's (1927) conditioned response ever actually flashed back to their acquisition experiences, the mechanism of classical conditioning is apparent in every case of PTSD. As salivation is to Pavlov's dog, so PTSD is to its victims.

Like emotional problems of other sorts, however, PTSD is not accounted for solely in terms of antecedent trauma and classical conditioning. In order to provoke a significant stress reaction, as Ellis (1962) and others observe, an experience must ordinarily stimulate certain components of an individual's pre-existing irrational beliefs. Veronen and Kilpatrick (1983) confirm that the rule holds for trauma as well as for more routine experience. Errant beliefs—related to the tolerance of discomfort and distress; performance, approval, and self-worth; and how others should behave—

> "…may be activated by traumatic events and lead to greater likelihood of developing and maintaining PTSD symptomatology and other emotional reactions. Individuals who pre-morbidly hold such beliefs in a dogmatic and rigid fashion are at greater risk of developing PTSD and experiencing more difficulty coping with the resulting PTSD symptomatology"
> (Warren & Zgourides, 1991, p. 151).

Also activated and often shattered by trauma are assumptions regarding personal invulnerability; a world that is meaningful, comprehensible, predictable and just; and the trustworthiness of others (Janoff-Bulman, 1985; Roth & Newman, 1991). Such pre-existing beliefs and assumptions, plus the various conclusions, decisions and attitudes specific to a particular traumatic incident (especially when held as imperatives) constitute the operant cognitive components of PTSD.

## Primary and Secondary Trauma

What makes PTSD a particularly persistent and pernicious variety of disturbance is the occurrence, at the time of its acquisition trauma, of significant physical and/or emotional pain. Such pain, in association with the other perceptual stimuli, thoughts, and feelings one experiences at the time, constitutes the "primary" traumatic incident. The composite memory of the primary incident, therefore, contains not only the dominant audio/visual impressions of that moment, but also one's mind-set (motives, purposes, intentions) and visceral (emotional and somatic) reactions. Thus, whenever one subsequently encounters a "restimulator"—any present-time sensory, perceptual, cognitive, or emotive stimulus similar to one of those contained in the memory of an earlier trauma—one is likely to be consciously or unconsciously "reminded" of and, therefore, to re-activate its associated pain or upset. It is this subsequent painful reminder, the involuntary "restimulation" of the primary trauma, that constitutes the painful secondary experience we recognize as PTSD (Foa, 1989).

In the Pavlovian model, the occurrence of the restimulator (trigger stimulus) equates to the ringing of the bell; the stress reaction itself equates to salivation. The mechanism is almost indefinitely extendible by association. Once the dog has been conditioned to salivate to the ringing of the bell, for example, the bell may be paired with a new perceptual stimulus—say, the flashing of a light—so that the dog will then salivate to the light as well as to the bell. If one next flashes the light and pulls the dog's tail, the dog will learn to salivate when his tail is pulled (Hilgard, 1962). By sequencing stimuli so as to create a "conditioned response chain" in this manner, we expand the domain of stimuli that will elicit the salivation response.

This process may be illustrated by the following common example: A veteran originally injured in an artillery attack (the primary trauma) will often tend to be restimulated, even years later, by such things as smoke and loud noises. So it's no surprise when he panics, post-war, in response to fireworks. However, should he happen to be triggered into a full-blown panic reaction by a fireworks display while eating fried chicken one day at a picnic in the park, he is likely thereafter, as strange as it seems, to get panicky around fried chicken (whether he flashes back to the park at the time or not). In such a circumstance, fried chicken gets added to the domain of toxic secondary restimulators of his war experience, and the "picnic in the park" incident acquires secondary trauma status and is itself subject to later restimulation. If, for instance, fried chicken subsequently gets (or previously had gotten) associated with his mother-in-law (who prepares it for his every visit), his contact with her also becomes subject to PTSD toxicity by association. The dynamic effect of such repeated reactions over a period of time is a gradual increase in the client's toxic secondary reactions. This, in turn, produces a corresponding reduction of his day-to-day rationality and an inability both to comprehend and to break out of his increasingly volatile reactive pattern (see Hayman et al, 1987).

The more reactions one experiences, the more new toxic secondary stimuli develop. The more new toxic stimuli there are, the more reactions one has, which suggests that those experiencing PTSD would eventually come to spend most of their time with their attention riveted painfully on past trauma. In point of fact, that does happen. The longer and more complex the chains or sequences of secondary incidents become over time, however, the less likely one is to flash all the way back to the primary trauma. This is why so many PTSD clients who appear to succeed in getting their attention off their primary traumata nevertheless withdraw from many of the life activities they previously enjoyed. Because they flash back to "the big one" a lot less, their PTSD cases are presumed to have abated. In reality such clients are in worse shape overall because a lot of little things in their traumatic incident networks (all the secondary restimulators or "cues" they picked up in the years following their primary traumata) bother them much more than they did in the past (Gerbode, 1995).

# PTSD and the Cognitive Therapies

Gerbode points out that some of the key cognitions contained in the memory of any traumatic incident that later cause trouble when they are restimulated are those specific conclusions, decisions, and intentions the individual generated during the incident itself in order to cope emotionally with the painful urgency of the moment. In such a circumstance, not only would certain pre-existing beliefs govern one's reaction to a traumatic event, but also the traumatic event itself would give rise to the formulation of new, potential errant cognitions. Viewed in this light, PTSD is very much a cognitive-emotive disorder and not nearly as Pavlovian as it at first appears to be. Accordingly, an effective cognitive-emotive approach is called for in its remediation, one in which the errant cognitions generated under the duress of the trauma are located and corrected.

Most cognitive therapists have traditionally favored challenging a client's current disturbance-causing belief system over directly confronting the earlier experience(s) responsible for its acquisition (Ellis, 1962, 1989). A therapist's decision to focus an intervention mainly on a client's responses to day-to-day stressors is most understandable when the client does not report flashing back at the time of the upsets. Most non-PTSD clients, after all, have no special awareness of their early acquisition experiences and, therefore, have little or nothing to say about them. Their attention is fixed on a steady stream of disturbance-provoking current events for which both we and they realize they do need more rational coping skills. In the clear-cut PTSD case in which flashback is evident, the client not only puts the acquisition experience (the primary trauma) in focus right at the start but also often seems virtually obsessed by it. Flashback content, which is often concurrent with the client's upset over something in present time, is so painfully "charged" that he or she is either barely able to shift attention from it or else must regularly struggle to resist attending to it (Solomon, 1991). In such a circumstance, the therapist who focuses intervention exclusively on the client's dramatic over-reactions to current (secondary) events (on the restimulator, rather than on what is being restimulated) bypasses the opportunity to address directly and resolve the core of the client's PTSD case. Such attention mainly to the present-time "cueing effect," according to Goodman and Maultsby (1974, p. 62), "explains many failures or partial successes in psychotherapy, despite the best intentions of patient and therapist."

Given the extreme volatility of the memory of a trauma, though, it's really no wonder that many therapists and their PTSD clients (tacitly) agree not to confront such incidents head on. To understand why this is so often the case, consider the following:

- It is nearly impossible to get PTSD clients to perceive or appraise objectively a traumatic experience they are in the midst of dramatizing;
- It is usually difficult, even when they are not dramatizing, to sell PTSD clients on the idea of re-evaluating a traumatic event that has given them nightmares for the last fifteen or twenty years;

- Cognitive restructuring, thought stopping, and stimulus blunting techniques give PTSD clients little or no control over their tendency to flashback spontaneously and go into restimulation; and

- Helping PTSD clients minimize the disruptive impact of their intrusive thoughts and teaching them not to down themselves over the persistence of their symptoms is better than nothing.

It becomes understandable, then, that many therapists choose to assist clients in their ongoing struggles to distance themselves from the memories of their traumata in an attempt simply to limit the frequency and intensity of their post-traumatic episodes.

Therapists may actually bring superb therapeutic skills to bear on clients' over-reactions to a variety of contemporary stimulus-events (e.g., rage over a spill, anxiety at a meeting), but unless they help PTSD clients to resolve the prior trauma (e.g., auto accident, childhood abuse, war experience) that actively supports their current disturbance and to revise the errant cognition associated with that primary experience, they have elected not to address the PTSD at all. The result of such a purely secondary intervention is that clients' unresolved primary traumas continue intermittently to intrude into consciousness, and clients are left to struggle alone to secure a sense of rationality against the influence of these traumas.

## Primary Approaches

Because a traumatic incident is, by definition, exceedingly unpleasant, there is an understandable tendency, at the moment one is occurring, to resist and protest it as best one can. It is at just such moments of extreme physical and/or emotional pain, according to Gerbode (1995), that one's thinking (evaluative cognition) is least likely to be well-reasoned and objective and most likely to be irrational and distorted. There is, moreover, a subsequent tendency to suppress and/or repress the memory of such an incident so as not to have to re-experience the painful emotional "charge" its restimulation carries with it. Unfortunately, suppression/repression of the memory of a traumatic incident effectively locks its distorted ideation and painful emotion away together (along with the incident's sensory and perceptual data) in long-term storage. Thus, the stage for PTSD is set. Fortunately however, when accessed with the specific cognitive imagery procedure of TIR, a primary traumatic incident can be stripped of its emotional charge permitting its embedded cognitive components to be revealed and restructured. With its emotional impact depleted and its irrational ideation revised, the memory of a traumatic incident becomes innocuous and thereafter remains permanently incapable of restimulation and intrusion into present time (Gerbode 1989).

As Manton and Talbot (1990) observe:

> "Traumatic events...can bring into consciousness unresolved [prior] situations (with similar themes) such as incest, child abuse, or the death of an important person in the victim's life" (p.508).

When clients have more than one trauma in their history, the only completely effective procedure is one that traces each symptom of the composite post-traumatic reaction back through sequence(s) of related earlier incidents to each of the contributing primaries. Interestingly, a very similar observation was made by one of our earliest colleagues, (Freud, 1984) who wrote:

> "What left the symptom behind was not always a single experience. On the contrary, the result was usually brought about by the convergence of several traumas, and often by the repetition of a great number of similar ones. Thus it was necessary to reproduce the whole chain of pathogenic memories in chronologic order, or rather in reversed order, the latest ones first and the earliest ones last" (p. 37).

The simple fact is that in order to deal effectively with past trauma, we must guide the client through to its resolution in imagery. The imagery process itself, however, is just the means by which we help PTSD clients get through their residual primary pain. It is by revising the errant cognition associated with that pain that they are freed from the grip of their PTSD.

## Traumatic Incident Reduction

The most thorough and reliable approach to the resolution of both long-standing and recent disaster PTSD currently in use is Traumatic Incident Reduction (TIR), a guided cognitive imagery procedure developed by Gerbode (1995). A high-precision refinement of earlier cognitive desensitization procedures, TIR effectively resolves the outstanding trauma of the majority of the PTSD clients with whom it is used when carried out according to its strict guidelines.

TIR appears to be more efficient and more effective than other cognitive-imagery or desensitization procedures, as such procedures frequently focus mainly (and most often incompletely) on secondary episodes. By tracing each traumatic reaction to its original or primary trauma(ta) and by taking each primary trauma to its full resolution or procedural "end point" at one sitting (a crucial requirement), the TIR process leaves clients observably relieved, often smiling, and no longer committed to their previously errant cognitions. At that point, the traumatic incidents, their associated irrational ideation, and consequent PTSD have been fully handled, and clients are able to re-engage life comfortably in ways they might not have been able to do since their original traumata.

Done one-on-one, the core TIR procedure may be completed in as little as twenty minutes or it may require two or three hours (average: 1.5 hrs) of "viewing" per incident. No procedure that is confined to the fifty-minute hour can be considered flexible enough to handle the average primary traumatic incident. The therapist needs to be willing to take the time necessary to guide the client back through the relevant trauma, carefully following TIR procedural guidelines, to permit the client to work through the painful memories of the experience in order to restructure its cognitive content as needed for full resolution.

Ideally, PTSD clients correctly identify their active primary incidents during intake. Clients who have regular flashbacks generally do this with ease. Such clients may be briefed on TIR the same day and, if not on psychoactive drugs, scheduled for viewing the next day. Their PTSD problems can often be alleviated within the week. It is not unusual for a TIR narrative procedure to resolve an "unoccluded" (obvious) primary traumatic incident in as little as two or three hours. Case resolution then would depend mainly on how many primary and secondary traumata needed to be addressed to restore full functioning.

More commonly, however, PTSD clients do not correctly identify all their active primary incidents at intake. A war veteran, for instance, may at first report with conviction that it all dates back to Vietnam; he's only had the problem since then, and that is the content of his flashbacks. Once he gets into it, however, he is sometimes surprised to discover that his wartime experience was actually secondary to some previously occluded or less memorable earlier trauma.

In chronic cases, including some phobias and panic disorders in which flashbacks are absent, clients often have no clue at intake as to where or when their reaction patterns were actually acquired. Although technically not classified as PTSD, many such clients have had a significant number of stressful experiences over the years. Yet they cannot, at first, identify any one incident as having been much more significant than any other. They are often thoroughly frustrated and discouraged, as well as genuinely baffled, about the persistence of their symptoms. Those among them who lead otherwise comfortable lives and seem not to think much less rationally, day-to-day, than the majority of the population frequently come to the usually erroneous conclusion that their problems must be genetic in origin ("run in the family"). (Needless to say, such cases are not resolved within the week.) They are not generally a problem for TIR, however, as they may be handled to resolution very adequately by the thematic approach, a variation of the narrative procedure. Thematic TIR does not require clients to be aware of or to identify correctly the relevant historic components of their cases right at the start of their intervention. Instead, the thematic procedure simply traces each manifest (present time) emotional and somatic symptom (theme) back through its chain(s) of secondary incidents, one at a time, until the originally occluded primaries come into awareness and can be dealt with routinely.

Toward clients' understanding of the TIR routine, which assuredly will be new to them, it is often useful to draw upon the illustrative value of the Pavlovian example mentioned earlier and with which they may already be familiar. One may point out, in this connection, that when the dog's salivation response to the bell (primary stimulus) is extinguished, the light (secondary stimulus) loses its restimulative potential automatically (Hilgard, 1962). Likewise, once a primary incident is completely resolved, none of the stimuli that had later become associated with it as secondary restimulators is capable of triggering any further reaction (Gerbode, 1989). This means that when the veteran fully resolves his "artillery attack" (and any other related primary incidents), he will no longer be vulnerable to restimulation triggered by the various secondarily toxic stimuli associated with that experience. At that point, fried chicken and mother-in-law are back to representing nothing more than fried chicken and mother-in-law.

This may seem like a rather classical Pavlovian explanation, but one of TIR's main concerns is the ultimate correction of the PTSD client's trauma-related thought processes. Once clients realize that it was the cumulative effect of their traumatic incident networks on their cognitive-emotive response sets over a period of time that is responsible for the persistence of their PTSD symptoms, and once they understand that there is a way to shut down the networks' active components permanently, they'll be happy to use the TIR approach, even if they are already accustomed to another technique. Then, even thoroughly frustrated and discouraged chronic and absent-flashback PTSD clients will begin to feel hopeful.

The lexicon of TIR reflects its purpose and procedure. The client is called a "viewer" because his/her primary function is to confront, via the viewing process, past trauma. The person conducting the session is called a "facilitator" because his/her purpose is simply to facilitate the viewer's process of viewing (Gerbode, 1989). Just as "physician" and "patient" become "analyst" and "analysand" or "surgeon" and "organ donor," based on the requirements of their respective roles, the designations "facilitator" and "viewer" are reserved for those whose interaction is governed by the singular requirements of the TIR process.

TIR, like other cognitive-imagery processes, differs somewhat from most contemporary therapies. Although it holds errant cognition to be at the root cause of emotional disturbance, unlike the mainstream cognitive approaches, TIR carries the revision process back to the specific experience(s) that originally produced and enforced such cognition. In this regard, TIR is a bit more "personal" than most contemporary cognitive therapies. Instead of relying mainly upon the therapist's insight into or inferences about a client's probable belief structure, as is common in Rational Emotive Behavioral Therapy (REBT), TIR guides clients in the discovery and revision of their own original disturbance-causing cognitions.

What makes such a procedure both necessary and possible is the fact that, in PTSD, the disturbance-causing cognitions (except for the pre-existing ones) were originally generated in response to, and in order to cope with, a traumatically painful and/or upsetting experience. Moreover, the offending cognitions are still being kept in force by the long-term residual impact of the incident. In other words, if it hadn't been for the specific circumstance of the trauma, as subjectively experienced by the client, e.g., "Oh my God, I've been shot! I'm gonna die!", the client wouldn't have formulated the response, e.g., "I should never let my guard down, even for a minute!" Moreover, if the incident hadn't been so emotionally and/or physically painful, making it extremely difficult for the client to confront, its attendant cognition would be a great deal more accessible to routine reappraisal and restructuring.

So, while it remains very useful to be able to infer with reasonable certainty that an anxious client is generally feeling threatened and ineffectual while an angry client would like to assert control over something (pardon the reductionism), these are just some of the more obvious "common denominator" dynamics associated with their respective current disturbances. What we cannot infer, but what TIR reveals to clients who have experienced trauma is exactly what happened (at a subjective/cognitive-emotive level) that so overwhelmed them that they would come away from their experience stuck in an involuntary, out-of-date, and irrational mind-set constructed, among other things, of numerous fairly obvious stress-producing mis-evaluations and distortions.

In a certain respect, TIR adds a new dimension to our understanding of the relationship between cognition and emotion. While theorists have long held that irrational thinking tends to promote upset feelings, TIR suggests that one's (traumatically) upset feelings also tend to promote irrational thinking. Dodging the "Which came first?" (chicken or egg) question, it is probably safe to say that, on the face of it, the causal equation appears to be reversible. That is, not only does cognition significantly influence emotion, but emotion appears to significantly influence cognition.

Even more critically significant, at least in cases of PTSD, the remedial equation seems to be reversible as well. Whereas cognitive therapists observe that the restructuring of one's irrational and distorted thinking produces a corresponding reduction of emotional disturbance, TIR confirms Ellis' (1990) observation that a reduction of primary traumatic emotional disturbance produces a corresponding restructuring of one's irrational and distorted thinking. In short, the client whose trauma has been fully reduced and resolved and who has become able to talk (and think) freely and painlessly about it (a TIR goal) almost immediately and self-directedly begins to display a substantively rational (moderate, tolerant, objective) viewpoint regarding that previously painful experience. As always, the client who succeeds in embracing a more rational viewpoint about an experience, regardless of how unfortunate or traumatic that experience once seemed, is no longer disturbed over it or unwittingly under its control. As a consequence, secondary restimulation and flashbacks cease, life's energy and interest revive, and self-esteem rebounds.

What is particularly remarkable about the cognitive restructuring that takes place in TIR is that it takes place so obviously and spontaneously during the course of a given session. Equally remarkable is the fact that it takes place—and truly must take place—without didactic or corrective facilitator input. The facilitator's role in TIR is mainly to so conduct the session and guide the viewer in "repeated review" of the selected trauma (in strict accord with the established protocol) that the viewer will be able rationally to restructure his own "misconceptions" about it (Raimy, 1975). Bear in mind that at this level of intervention the viewer is truly the only one who can decipher (by patient and careful re-examination of the cognitive images stored in memory) what actually happened or appeared to happen in the incident, what its significance was, what he or she was thinking at the time, why it was so extraordinarily painful, how he or she coped with that pain, and what trauma-related conclusions and/or decisions were made at the time. So, as the viewer reviews this highly sensitive and very painful material repeatedly in imagery in order to discharge the emotional impact holding the cognitive distortions in place, the facilitator says not a word.

Although in TIR's handling of PTSD the operant trauma-related distortions virtually self-correct once the inordinate emotional distress of the traumatic experience is relieved, viewers frequently want to follow a completed TIR session with some discussion or review of some of the ways in which certain of their newly surrendered trauma-related beliefs and attitudes had affected them since the occurrence of their original trauma. Most practitioners find this discussion one of those truly rewarding moments in clinical practice. It is not only confirmation of a successfully completed specific intervention. It is re-confirmation of what contemporary theorists have asserted all along about the relationship between cognition and emotion—with the additional suggestion that that relationship may be even more interesting than we had originally supposed.

A fully resolved traumatic experience is neither completely nor mostly forgotten. It is, by definition, simply benign and incapable of intrusive restimulation.

## Bibliography

American Psychiatric Association (1987). Diagnostic and statistical manual of mental disorders (3rd edit.), Revised, APA, Washington, D.C.

Beck, A. T. (1970). Role of fantasies in psychotherapy and psychopathology. The Journal of Nervous and Mental Disease, 150, 3-17.

Beck, A. T. (1976). Cognitive therapy and the emotional disorders. New York: The New American Library, Inc.

Blundell, G. G., and Cade, C. M. (1980). Self-awareness and E.S.R. London: Audio Ltd.

Boudewyns, P. A., Hyer, L., Woods, M. G., Harrison, W. R., and McCranie, E. (1990). PTSD among Vietnam veterans: An early look at treatment outcome using direct therapeutic exposure. Journal of Traumatic Stress, 3, 359-368.

Dansky, B. S., Roth, S., and Kronenberger, W. G. (1990). The trauma constellation identification scale: A measure of the psychological impact of a stressful life event. J. of Traumatic Stress, 3, 557-572.

Dryden, W., and Ellis, A. (1986). Rational-emotive therapy (RET). In W. Dryden and W. Golden (Eds.), Cognitive-behavioral approaches to psychotherapy. London: Harper & Row.

Ellis, A. (1962). Reason and emotion in psychotherapy. New York: Lyle Stuart.

Ellis, A. (1973). Humanistic psychotherapy: The rational-emotive approach. New York: McGraw Hill.

Ellis, A. (1989). The history of cognition in psychotherapy. In A. Freeman, K. M. Simon, L. E. Beutler, and H.

Arkowitz (Eds.), Comprehensive handbook of cognitive therapy (pp. 5-19). New York: Plenum Publishing.

Ellis, A. (1990). The revised ABC's of rational-emotive therapy (RET). Paper presented at The Evolution of Psychotherapy conference, Anaheim, CA.

Eth, S., and Pynoos, R. S. (Eds.). (1985). Posttraumatic stress disorder in children. Washington, D.C.: American Psychiatric Press.

Fairbank, J. A., and Nicholson, R. A. (1987). Theoretical and empirical issues in the treatment of post-traumatic stress disorder in Vietnam veterans. Journal of Clinical Psychology, 43, 44-55.

Foa, E. B., and Olasov, B. (1989). Treatment of post-traumatic stress disorder. Workshop conducted at Advances in Theory and Treatment of Anxiety Disorders, Philadelphia, PA.

Foa, E. B., Steketee, G., and Rothbaum, B. O. (1989). Behavioral-cognitive conceptualizations of post-traumatic stress disorder. Behavior Therapy, 20, 155-176.

Frederick, C. J. (1986, August) Psychic trauma and terrorism. Paper presented at the annual meeting of the American Psychological Association, Washington, D.C.

French, G. D. (1991). Traumatic incident reduction workshop manual. Menlo Park, CA: IRM.

Freud, S. (1984). Two short accounts of psychoanalysis. In J. Strachey (Tr.), Five lectures on psychoanalysis (p. 37). Singapore: Penguin Books.

Gerbode, F. A. (1986a). Assistance without evaluation. The Journal of Metapsychology, 1, 7-9.

Gerbode, F. A. (1986b). A safe space. The J. of Metapsychology, 1, 3-6.

Gerbode, F. A. (1995). Beyond psychology: An introduction to Metapsychology (3rd Ed).. Palo Alto, CA: IRM.

Goodman, D. S. and Maultsby, M. C. (1974). Emotional well-being through rational behavior training. Springfield, IL: Charles C. Thomas.

Grossberg, J. M., and Wilson, H. K. (1968). Physiological changes accompanying the visualization of fearful and neutral situations. Journal of Personality and Social Psychology, 10, 124-133.

Hayman, P. M., Sommers-Flanagan, R., and Parsons, J. P. (1987). Aftermath of violence: Post-traumatic stress disorder among Vietnam veterans. Journal of Counseling and Development, 65, 363-366.

Hilgard, E. R. (1962). Introduction to psychology (3rd Edition). New York: Harcourt, Brace & World, Inc.

Horowitz, M. (1986). Stress Response Syndromes (2nd ed.). Northvale, NJ: Jason Aronson.

Janoff-Bulman R. (1985). The aftermath of victimization: Rebuilding shattered assumptions. In C. R. Figley (Ed.), Trauma and its wake. New York: Brunner/Mazel.

Keane, T. M., and Kaloupek, D. G. (1982). Imaginal flooding in the treatment of a posttraumatic stress disorder. Journal of Consulting and Clinical Psychology, 50, 138-140.

Keane, T. M., Fairbank, J. A., Caddell, J. M., and Zimering, R. T. (1989). Implosive (flooding) therapy reduces symptoms of PTSD in Vietnam combat veterans. Behavior Therapy, 20, 245-260.

Kelly, W. E. (Ed.). (1985). Post-traumatic stress disorder and the war veteran patient. New York: Brunner/Mazel.

# Psychological Foundations of TIR
## By Robert H. Moore, Ph.D.

## Introduction

Developed by Frank A. Gerbode, M.D. TIR is a regressive desensitization procedure for reducing or eliminating the negative residual impact of traumatic experience. As such it finds major application in cases of post-traumatic stress disorder (PTSD). A one-on-one guided imagery process, TIR is also useful in remediation of specific unwanted stress responses, such as panic attacks, that occur without significant provocation. "Thematic TIR" traces such conditioned responses back through the history of their occurrence in a client's life to the stressful incidents primarily responsible for their acquisition. The resolution of the primary incidents then reduces or eliminates the target stress response.

As an intervention technique, TIR is both directive and client-centered. It is directive in that the therapist who is called a "facilitator" guides the client who is called a "viewer" repetitively through an imaginal replay of a specific trauma. It is client—or, as Dr. Gerbode prefers, "person-" - centered, in that a TIR facilitator doesn't interpret or critique the viewer's experience or tell him how he should feel or what to think about it. A methodical and systematic anamnesis, TIR unsuppresses the trauma being addressed to provide the viewer the opportunity to review and revise his perspective on it. TIR's uniqueness lies, in part, in the fact that a session continues until the viewer is completely relieved of whatever stress the target trauma originally provoked and any cognitive distortions (e.g., observations, decisions, conclusions) embedded within the incident have been restructured. (Gerbode, 1989)

## TIR's Philosophic Roots

TIR and virtually every other contemporary regressive and imaginal desensitization procedure used in the remediation of trauma—including "sequential analysis" (Blundell and Cade), "direct therapeutic exposure" (Boudewyns), "prolonged imaginal exposure" (Foa and Olasov), "gradual dosing" (Horowitz), "flooding" (Keane and Kaloupek), "repetitive review" (Raimy), and "implosion" (Stampfl and Lewis)—derive directly from principles clearly articulated in the earliest writings of Freud and Pavlov. Although the latter, Pavlov, is properly credited with the identification of the "conditional reflex" and its chain-linked "secondary signaling system" (the model most commonly referenced in connection with PTSD acquisition), Freud earlier had made the equivalent observation about the development of the traumatic neuroses. He wrote:

> What left the symptom behind was not always a single experience. On the contrary, the result was usually brought about by the convergence of several traumas, and often by the repetition of a great number of similar ones. Thus it was necessary to reproduce the whole chain of pathogenic memories in chro-

nologic order, or rather in reversed order, the latest ones first and the earliest ones last. (1984, p. 37)

The essential congruity of the Pavlovian and Freudian observations, in this connection, prompted Astrup (1965) to note that:

> From a conditional reflex point of view, psychoanalytic therapy represents a continuous association experiment with subtle analysis of second signaling system connections... (p. 126)

As TIR draws heavily on these same well-established principles, Dr. Gerbode, who was originally schooled in psychoanalysis, and Dr. Robert H. Moore—a cognitive-behaviorist colleague, and author of these notes—routinely reference this intersection of the Freudian and Pavlovian constructs in presentations of TIR to the mental health professions.

## PTSD And Imaginal Procedures

Whether favoring the remedial logic of "abreaction" or of "extinction," dedicated trauma workers display a strong and growing philosophic and clinical consensus regarding the importance of addressing traumatic experience with a guided imagery procedure like that employed by TIR.

In their review of theoretical and empirical issues in the treatment of PTSD, Fairbank and Nicholson (1987) conclude that, of all the approaches in use, only those involving some form of direct imaginal exposure to the trauma have been successful.

Roth and Newman (1991) describe the ideal resolution process as one involving "a re-experiencing of the affect associated with the trauma in the context of painful memories." Such a process, the authors point out, brings the individual "to both an emotional and cognitive understanding of the meaning of the trauma and the impact it has had...and would lead to a reduction in symptoms and to successful integration of the trauma experience" (p. 281).

Grossberg and Wilson (1968) have shown that repeated visualization of a fearful situation produces a significant drop in the physiological response [Galvanic Skin Response or GSR] to the threatening image.

Folkins, Lawson, Opton, and Lazarus (1968) have demonstrated the efficacy of rehearsal in fantasy in reducing the physiological response (GSR) to a frightening movie.

Blundell and Cade (1980) independently confirm that repeated visualization of an anxiety-provoking situation produces a significant reduction in the physiological (GSR) response to the threatening image. Frederick (1986) used a very TIR-like desensitization procedure with trauma victims:

He contended that such incident-specific treatment is essential to overcoming PTSD. Using mental images, the client reviews, frame by frame, the entire sequence of the traumatic experience. During the process, the client is able to recall and disclose significant thoughts and feelings related to the trauma and, consequently, anxiety associated with the trauma dissipates. (Hayman, Sommers-Flanagan, and Parsons, 1987)

R. D. Laing concurs:

> You can look at it with such narcissistic bonding as to bring tears to your eyes, or grimaces of distaste at what you see. After each paroxysm of self-pity or self-disgust or self-adulation, look at it again and again, and again until those tears are dry, the laughter has subsided, the sobs have ceased. Then look at it, quite dispassionately ...until you've got nothing to do with it at all. (Russell and Laing, 1992)

Some trauma therapists employ hypnosis as an accessing tool. Although this is not the case in TIR, it is interesting to note the similarity of the hypnotic and non-hypnotic approaches to resolution, once the client has contacted and begun to unsuppress a traumatic incident.

The Ericksonian procedure for addressing the content of a traumatic incident employs a trance state. Following hypnotic induction, his retrospective "jigsaw" technique guides the client in recovery of the cognitive and emotive components of a painful memory in whatever order the client can most easily confront:

> Various bits of the incident recovered in this jigsaw fashion allow you to eventually recover an entire, forgotten traumatic experience of childhood that had been governing this person's behavior...and handicapping his life very seriously. (Erickson, 1955/80)

MacHovec (1985) confirms that hypnotic regression can be used to help clients recall and revivify a traumatic incident, vent emotions, and gradually reintegrate the experience with improved coping skills.

## PTSD And Cognitive Restructuring

Like other effective trauma resolution processes, TIR is not primarily a cathartic technique. Gerbode (1986) affirms the professional consensus that cognitive restructuring is prerequisite for thorough trauma resolution. Raimy (1975) concurs:

> Many current therapies attempt primarily to relieve the client or patient of his pent-up emotion, either in cathartic episodes or over longer periods of time in which emotional release takes place less dramatically. If we examine catharsis more closely, however, we can readily discover several cognitive events which have significant influence on the experience. If these cognitive events do not occur, no amount of "emotional expression" is likely to be helpful (p. 81).

Speaking specifically to the use of imaginal exposure in the rational-emotive treatment of PTSD, Warren and Zgourides (1991) report that:

Keane et al's (1989) implosive therapy, Horowitz's (1986) gradual dosing, and Foa and Olasov's (1987) prolonged imaginal exposure are methods that help clients work through their traumatic event, discover and revise meanings, and develop more adaptive responses to the traumatic event. In RET [Rational Emotive Behavioral Therapy], we incorporate imaginal exposure to the traumatic event.. (and).. While conducting the imaginal exposure and in reviewing imagined and behavioral exposure homework assignments, we are on the lookout for clients' cognitive and emotional reprocessing of the trauma that may relate to the issues of meaning of the event, shattered assumptions, irrational beliefs, and so on. (p. 161)

Beck (1970) lends additional support to the importance of cognitive restructuring during what he calls "rehearsals in fantasy" in his observation that:

When a patient has an unpleasant affect associated with a particular situation, the unpleasant affect may sometimes be eliminated or reduced with repeated imagining of the situation even though the content of the fantasy does not change. The unpleasant affect may be shame, sadness, anxiety, or disgust.

The data collected from patients and these experimental studies suggest that the rehearsals in fantasy produce a cognitive restructuring. With each voluntary repetition of the fantasy, the patient is enabled to discriminate more sharply between real dangers and purely imaginary or remote dangers. As he is able to appraise the fantasy more realistically, the threat and the accompanying anxiety are reduced.

Through fantasy induction (the client) is able to recognize the specific details of his conception of the situation, to reality-test this conception, and to correct the distortions. The standard techniques of free association or direct discussion of the problem may fail to illuminate the conceptualization, whereas the fantasy expression brings it into sharp focus. Once the distorted picture has been corrected, the patient feels better and can handle the situation more efficiently.

## Training

Successful clinical application of TIR requires a minimum of four days of intensive training—which includes skill development exercises, live and videotaped demonstration sessions, and both giving and receiving TIR sessions under the supervision of a trainer certified by the Association (see www.TIR.org)—followed by an optional practicum with consultation.

## References

Astrup, C. (1965). Pavlovian psychiatry: a new synthesis. Springfield, IL: Charles C. Thomas.

Beck, A. T. (1970). "Role of fantasies in psychotherapy and psychopathology". The Journal of Nervous and Mental Disease, 150, 3-17.

Blundell, G. G., and Cade, C. M. (1980). Self-awareness and E.S.R. London: Audio Ltd.

Boudewyns, P. A., Hyer, L., Woods, M. G., Harrison, W. R., and McCranie, E. (1990). "PTSD among Vietnam veterans: An early look at treatment outcome using direct therapeutic exposure." Journal of Traumatic Stress, 3, 359-368.

Erickson, M. (1955/80). Self-exploration in the hypnotic state. In E. Rossi (Ed.), The collected papers of Milton H. Erickson on Hypnosis. Vol IV. Innovative Hypnotherapy (427-436). New York: Irvington.

Fairbank, J. A., and Nicholson, R. A. (1987). Theoretical and empirical issues in the treatment of post-traumatic stress disorder in Vietnam veterans. Journal of Clinical Psychology, 43, 44-55.

Foa, E. B., and Olasov, B. (1989). "Treatment of post-traumatic stress disorder." Workshop conducted at Advances in Theory and Treatment of Anxiety Disorders, Philadelphia, PA.

Folkins, C. H., Lawson, K. D., Opton, E. M., and Lazarus, R.S. (1968). "Desensitization and the experimental reduction of threat." Journal of Abnormal Psychology, 73, 100-113.

Frederick, C. J. (1986, August) Psychic trauma and terrorism. Paper presented at the annual meeting of the American Psychological Association, Washington, D.C.

French, G. D. (1991). Traumatic Incident Reduction Workshop Manual. Menlo Park, CA: IRM.

Freud, S. (1984). Two short accounts of psychoanalysis. In J. Strachey (Tr.), Five lectures on psychoanalysis (p. 37). Singapore: Penguin Books.

Gerbode, F. A. (1986). Indicators and end points. The Journal of Metapsychology, 1, 51-56.

Gerbode, F. A. (1989). Beyond Psychology: an Introduction to Metapsychology. Menlo Park, CA: IRM.

Grossberg, J. M., and Wilson, H. K. (1968). Physiological changes accompanying the visualization of fearful and neutral situations. Journal of Personality and Social Psychology, 10, 124-133.

Hayman, P. M., Sommers-Flanagan, R., and Parsons, J. P. (1987). Aftermath of violence: post-traumatic stress disorder among Vietnam veterans. Journal of Counseling and Development, 65, 365.

Horowitz, M. (1986). Stress Response Syndromes (2nd ed.). Northvale, NJ: Jason Aronson.

Keane, T. M., Fairbank, J. A., Caddell, J. M., and Zimering, R. T. (1989). Implosive (flooding) therapy reduces symptoms of PTSD in Vietnam combat veterans. Behavior Therapy, 20, 245-260.

Keane, T. M., and Kaloupek, D. G. (1982). Imaginal flooding in the treatment of a posttraumatic stress disorder. Journal of Consulting and Clinical Psychology, 50, 138-140.

Lyons, J. A., and Keane, T. M. (1989). Implosive therapy for the treatment of combat-related PTSD. Journal of Traumatic Stress, 2, 137-152.

MacHovec, F. J. (1985). Treatment variables and the use of hypnosis in the brief therapy of post traumatic stress disorders. International Journal of Clinical & Experimental Hypnosis, 33, 6-14.

Manton, M., and Talbot, A. (1990). Crisis intervention after an armed hold-up: Guidelines for counselors. Journal of Traumatic Stress, 3, 507-22.

Moore, R. H. (1993). Traumatic incident reduction: a cognitive-emotive treatment of post-traumatic stress disorder. In W. Dryden and L. Hill (Eds.) Innovations in Rational-Emotive Therapy. Newbury Park, CA: Sage.

Pavlov, I. P. (1927). Conditioned reflexes. New York: Oxford Univ. Press.

Raimy, V. (1975). Misunderstandings of the self. San Francisco: Jossey-Bass Publishers.

Roth, S., and Newman, E. (1991). The process of coping with sexual trauma. Journal of Traumatic Stress, 4, 279-297.

Russell, R., and Laing R. D. (1992). R.D. Laing & me: Lessons in love. Lake Placid, NY: Hillgarth Press.

Stampfl, T. G., and Lewis, D. J. (1967). Essentials of implosive therapy: A learning-theory-based psychodynamic behavioral therapy. Journal of Abnormal Psychology, 72, 496-503.

Turner, S. M. (1979). Systematic desensitization of fears and anxiety in rape victims. Paper presented at the annual meeting of the Assoc. for the Advancement of Behavior Therapy, San Francisco, CA.

Warren, R., and Zgourides, G. D. (1991). Anxiety disorders: A rational-emotive perspective. Elmsford, NY: Pergamon.

# No Longer a Victim:

## A Treatment Outcome Study for Crime Victims with PTSD
## By Lori Beth Bisbey, Ph.D.

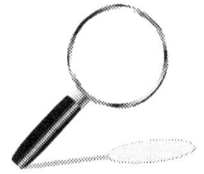

**2**

*The following transcript is excerpted from the plenary session of Lori Beth Bisbey, Ph.D. at the 8th Annual Conference on Metapsychology in 1994.*

As of 1994, the published research on PTSD primarily supported the use of relaxation and exposure-based techniques. One of the issues that has been raised by practitioners in connection with using these kinds of techniques, such as flooding, is the possibility that current trauma might be connected with earlier trauma. Does flooding address this issue? The implication is that any treatment which has both an exposure element and an element that deals with earlier trauma should be more successful in treating PTSD.

My study had three conditions.

One was Direct Therapeutic Exposure (DTE), which combined imaginal flooding and progressive relaxation. DTE protocol starts and ends with progressive muscle relaxation with flooding in-between. There is research indicating that this is a good way of doing it. For most people, flooding involves visual imagery, but not necessarily so, because some people are not visually based. Relaxation may improve the ability to visualize.

The second experimental condition was Traumatic Incident Reduction, the third a control group. We wanted to see which one (if either) treatment would be the more successful in treating crime victims who had PTSD. Before this study, there had been a lack of controlled outcome research with a sufficiently large population in this area. The first objective of this study was to provide a sound, sufficiently large treatment outcome experiment comparing a method that has been researched previously (DTE) to an upcoming method (TIR). These are the limitations of the previous research: small sample sizes, poor measures or instrumentation, multiple concurrent treatments, poor reporting and analysis of the demographic data, and poor inclusion and exclusion criteria. These are the issues that we tried to address when the study was constructed.

The second objective was to provide further data on the efficacy of DTE in treating a complex syndrome and to compare it with TIR. The third objective was to improve on these methodological flaws of the past. My study had 57 subjects, which is quite large in treatment outcome research, although it might sound small to you. It's the third largest study done on PTSD before 1995. In addition, what we did (myself and my committee), was to base our sample size on statistical power. I wanted to be sure that I would detect a difference between TIR and DTE if there was one. Also, earlier research often had poor inclusion and exclusion criteria. This meant that it wasn't clearly defined who were eligible for the research and therefore what population were you looking at. In my study, people were excluded on the basis of a diagnosis of active substance abuse, or if they did not qualify for a diagnosis of PTSD. We did not try to diagnose any other psychological or psychiatric disorder. This proved to be quite interesting.

We gathered detailed demographic data including subjects' previous experience in treatment. Another frequent issue is that a proportion of victims of crime and a proportion of people who suffer PTSD after an event get better on their own in three months, no matter what you do with them. I wanted to make sure that whatever results we got, it wasn't going to be able to be said that "Well, it was because that all of them were less than three months from the trauma." I'm not going to provide detailed demographics in this presentation, but people who are interested can obtain a reprint of my thesis from Dissertation Express [See Appendix A].

## Hypotheses

There were ten hypotheses for this study. The first three predicted that the treatment groups would show a significant decrease in PTSD-related symptom measures. The next two predicted that both treatment groups would show a larger decrease on two of the measures than the control group. Another hypothesis predicted that the treatment groups would show a decrease on an individual trauma checklist. There was one hypothesis that predicted that the TIR group would show a larger decrease in symptoms on that checklist. That was the only hypothesis that specifically compared the two treatments. The last group of hypotheses had to do with job and relationship satisfaction.

All the subjects were victims of crime. We didn't set out to choose people who were victims of just one crime or many crimes. As it turned out, 82.2% of the subjects were victims of violent crimes and 71.9% of the subjects were victims of more than one crime; that was from a random sample. Analysis using a lot of statistics showed up no demographic differences between the three groups. One factor showed up a difference that approached significance. I'll describe this later.

Concurrent treatment is one of the things that is frequently mentioned as a confounding problem in a research study of this type. It's not unusual to have someone referred for specific PTSD treatment who is already in therapy with somebody else, or to be on one or two different medications, or to be an inpatient. That's one of the areas that I looked at. There was one subject in the TIR group and two subjects in the DTE group who were on anti-depressant medication. They had all been on medication for more than three months prior to the study. None of my subjects were in any other type of treatment during the study and all of them had stopped other treatments at least three months prior.

There were four therapists, two men and two women (including myself). All were trained in both treatment methods, regardless of their previous training or experience. The purpose of this was to standardize their training. We did not look at gender differences between therapists. Whenever possible, subjects were pre- and post-tested by someone other than the primary therapist. Treatment subjects were randomly assigned to groups and given a maximum of twenty hours of treatment. First we looked at whether or not they were in relationships. We wanted to maximize the number of people across the groups who were in relationships so we could get relationship satisfaction data. Then they were randomly assigned. Treatment lasted approximately five weeks; we then post-tested two weeks later (at seven weeks).

The reason I say "approximately" in places is because, as you may know, TIR doesn't have a fixed session time. The DTE session groups were two hours each twice a week. For TIR, it didn't necessarily work out that way. Statistical analysis after the fact showed that this did not have a discriminating impact. The average total treatment times weren't significantly different. I found that people who had fewer treatment hours were actually doing better, which sounds strange. But, in fact when you look at, it does really make sense. People who had fewer treatment hours were possibly doing better to begin with. However, the difference was not statistically significant. The variation was very small, the typical subject having from 12 to 20 hours (average 17.9 hours) treatment.

I used a number of measures: the Penn Inventory (Hammerberg 1982), and the Impact of Events Scale (Horowitz, Wilner, & Alvarez, 1979) for PTSD. I used the Symptom Checklist (1990 revised) which has an embedded scale within it called the Crime-Related PTSD Scale. I used individual trauma checklists in which I took each trauma that the person reported and had them rate level of distress on a scale of 0 to 5. I used the work and co-worker scale from the Job Descriptive Index (JDI) to measure job satisfaction and the Dyadic Adjustment Scale for relationship satisfaction. I also used the Therapy Gain Scale because the therapists were doing a portion of each group and I needed to see if they were perceived differently depending on the treatment they were administering. No difference was shown there.

## Results

The TIR group performed better than DTE on the Impact of Events Scale (Fig. 1). This turned out in statistical tests to be quite significant. I used multivariate analysis of variance and followed that with extremely stringent criteria to make sure that if there was a difference between the groups that it wouldn't be an artifact. In this case, the TIR group was significantly different from DTE and both groups were significantly different from the control group. The Crime-Related PTSD Scale (Fig. 2) has a clear delineation between PTSD diagnosis and no diagnosis. What ended up happening was that more than 50% of all the treatment subjects no longer had PTSD. The TIR group was significantly different from the DTE group. The Penn Inventory also has a cutoff score and also showed TIR significantly different from DTE and the control groups.

What does all this mean? One of the things that didn't happen was differences in the relationship variables, which was somewhat surprising. However, we didn't really have enough subjects to see significant differences. Although we had 57 subjects, not all were in relationships that could be measured by this scale. The Dyadic Adjustment Scale measures relationships that are "serious" meaning that they are living together or married. We had many other people involved in relationships that were not that long-standing. Additionally, some of the subjects actually were in what they perceived to be negative relationships at the beginning of treatment. They saw that as a very positive change, but on the Dyadic Adjustment Scale it doesn't come out that way.

The same was true with job satisfaction. First, my choice of a measure was not very good, because people had difficulty understanding it. There were adjectives that they had to mark as "yes" or "no" about their job and co-workers. I chose this instrument because it had some standardization and I wanted to make sure it would relate to other areas. However, many people complained about it. Additionally we had the problem of not enough people again. Some people were unemployed at the start, some people quit their jobs during treatment, and still others found new jobs during the course of the study.

In hindsight, if I were to do this again, I would try to find different ways of measuring relationships and job satisfaction. One of the things said about TIR is that it affects more than just PTSD. This was the reason I wanted to look at other areas quantitatively and ask the question, "What other areas of life would successful TIR affect?" Unfortunately, I wasn't able to get this information. However, some very tentative supplementary analyses were done on a few of the nine sub-scales of the Symptom Checklist (1990 revised). The depression sub-scale was examined because it's one of the most common co-diagnoses that go along with PTSD. Interestingly enough, there was a significant difference between DTE and TIR vs. the control group.

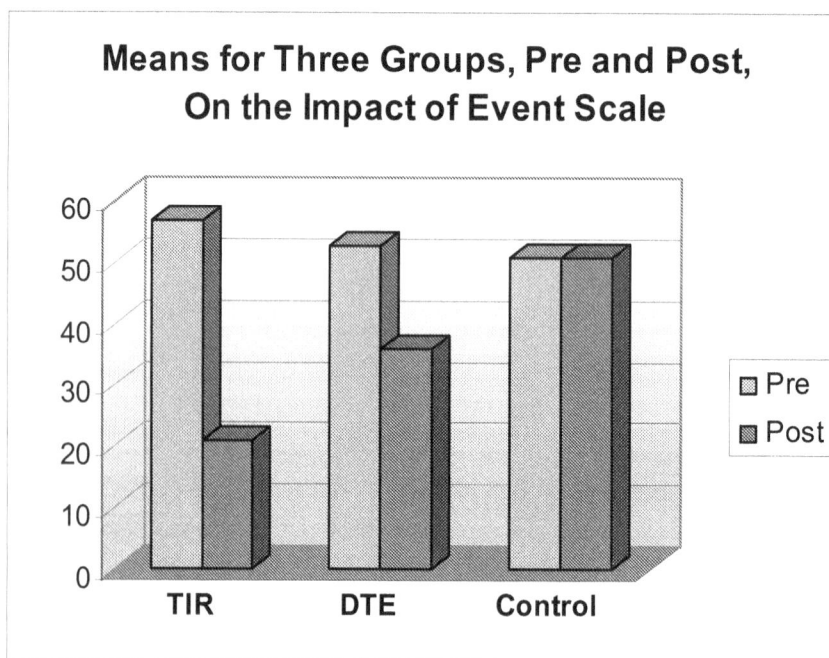

Impact of Events Scale (Fig. 1)

## Means for Three Groups, Pre and Post, On the Crime-Related PTSD Scale

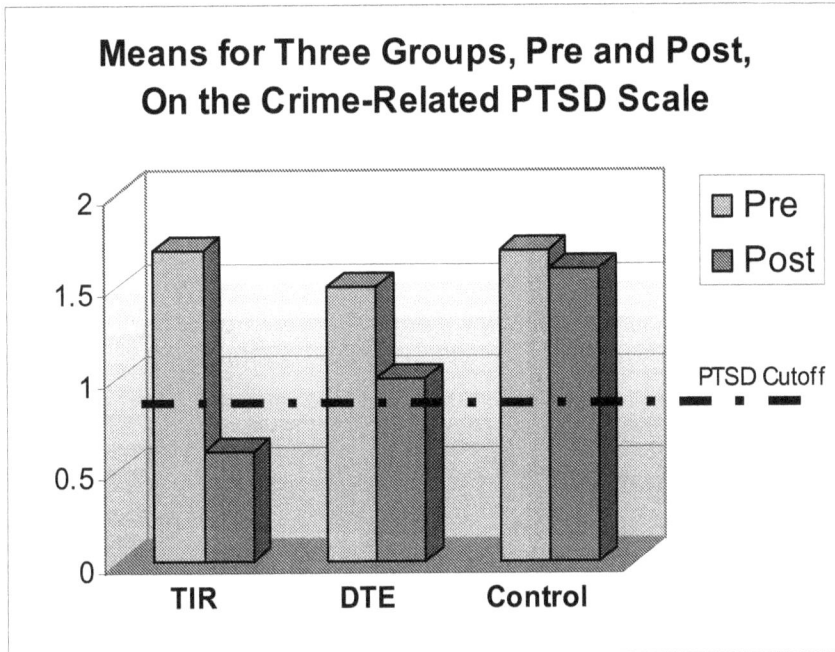

Crime-Related PTSD Scale (Fig. 2)

## Means for Three Groups, Pre and Post, On the Penn Inventory

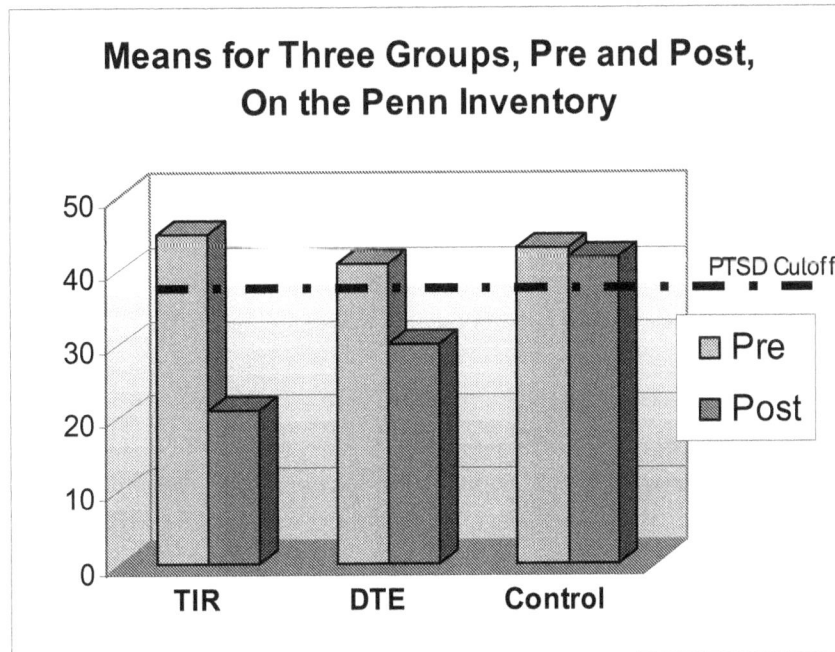

Penn Inventory (Fig. 3)

However, there was not a significance difference between the two treatment conditions. We weren't using the best measure of depression because it wasn't a central concern of the study and we didn't diagnose for it. I think the Beck scale would have given us a better pre/post measure. These were just reported depression symptoms and it's possible that if we diagnosed we might have found out that in some cases the depression was secondary to the PTSD and in other cases the depression preceded the PTSD. Those groups might look differently in terms of treatment effect (if they could have been isolated that way).

I wasn't actually looking at curing depression, but I was interested in the fact that depression results changed. Differences were maintained at six and twelve months' follow-up for people who had large differences. The TIR group is looking brilliant for the 6 months and 12 months results that we have. Nobody has gotten worse and nobody has relapsed. There are some people where things stayed the same and some people where things have gotten better.

A crucial issue to me is whether the person was already depressed and then traumatized or whether they were traumatized and the depression was a result of the trauma. It is possible that the treatments for PTSD affected depression for people who were not depressed before suffering trauma. We actually had a mixed bag; some people would have already had a diagnosis of depression before the trauma. Those people were probably the ones who didn't change. The implications of this are pretty important to patients in the UK. If you complain of PTSD and depression and you go to your family doctor, then you are prescribed anti-depressants. However, if they could actually distinguish which came first, the depression or the trauma, and then made an appropriate referral they would have a better resolution without having to medicate.

The Penn Inventory (Fig. 3) showed that after TIR, 89.47% no longer qualified for a diagnosis of PTSD. The corresponding figure for DTE was a pretty healthy 57.89%. In the control group, 31.58% had actually changed without intervention.

The other thing that changed was obsessive-compulsive symptoms. There is some suggestion that there is actually a relationship between some of these symptoms and PTSD.

The only other changes I noted on Symptom Checklist 90 was that the paranoid scale showed changes for both treatment groups; and the psychoticism scale changed for TIR but not for DTE. I didn't look at these specifically enough to give an adequate explanation. I propose that the next study looks for more than PTSD, and explores what other co-diagnoses might be present (using something other than the Symptom Checklist-90). I would suggest the Minnesota Multiphasic Personality Inventory-2 because I think that's a better measure of general psychopathology. My study was unable to answer the question of whether TIR is affecting things other than PTSD.

The study provides further evidence that exposure-based treatments or treatments that require repetitive contact with the trauma are very effective in treating PTSD. In previous research and theoretical articles, two factors have been hypothesized to be necessary for successful treatment: (1) exposure to the traumatic material (which both treatments obviously have) and (2) some sort of cognitive shift where the traumatized individual doesn't see the importance of the event in the same way. One of the criticisms frequently made about DTE-based treatments is that a cognitive shift occurs by luck rather than by design, if at all. In contrast, in TIR, specific questions may be used to actually provoke that cognitive shift. Personally, I think this is one explanation why the TIR group did better than the DTE group. I think the second explanation would be the issue of looking at earlier connected incidents, which DTE doesn't do and TIR does. There was some anecdotal evidence to support this. A couple of subjects completed DTE, and after post-testing were changed to TIR. These individuals had many, many traumas that were connected and knew that they were connected. They did much better with TIR than with DTE.

It is always possible that therapist bias and experience could have been responsible for the difference. Two of the four therapists were more experienced in TIR than in DTE; two of us had about equal experience in each. We tried to control for bias in this study by first of all standardizing the training of therapists before they participated in this study. Second, we added the Therapy Gain Scale to look at whether the therapists were perceived differently in treatments when they were doing DTE or TIR. No significant difference was found. We also had some external supervision on random samples of sessions to look at whether the sessions were being conducted properly. But even with all that, I think you can't completely control whether there was a bias in the research. After the issue was raised at my thesis defense, I went back and did further statistical analyses to see whether or not this was an issue. I believe the only way that this question will be answered is by replication (of the study).

What we do know is that both treatments work and that is an important message. For me, the highest significance is that DTE is the most researched treatment with PTSD to date. What we've learned as a result of this research is that TIR is at least as effective as DTE, and maybe more effective than DTE with this population. Our results show TIR to be significantly more effective, but we need to wait for replication because there hasn't been enough research on TIR. Still, my study is a good starting point; it's a good way to compare the results with what's already been done. We are gathering six-month, twelve-month, and two-year data and hopefully I'll report on that when it's finally collated. So far, both groups look like they are OK. So far, a few DTE subject have suffered partial relapses, but not one TIR subject has done so. We have collected more data on TIR subjects.

I have five definite one-year follow-ups on TIR subjects right now and I should say that these were complex cases. One of the interesting things was that it didn't matter how complex the case was in terms of hours. Some of the more complex cases took fewer hours to handle and that's quite strange. These were spectacular cases in that they had no symptoms left afterwards. After one year they were still at the same level, but there was intervening trauma. The comments I got back on the follow-up were:

> "This [crime] happened to me and it was amazing to see that I didn't react. I had a response to what was going on in the *present* and not what was triggered in the past."

That's been repeated and that's what's so exciting for me. That's why I want to keep collecting data as time goes on. What they're saying is: "I had a similar trauma, and I *did* react to it like any human being would react to it, but what didn't happen was that it didn't trigger earlier stuff and therefore it was resolvable quite easily on my own without needing intervention." To me that's not remission, although I do dislike the terms remission/non-remission in that model. That would actually be cure if they're not actually triggering into earlier stuff.

# From Psychology to Metapsychology: a Clinician's Journey

## by Lori Beth Bisbey, Ph.D.

*The following transcript is excerpted from the plenary session of Lori Beth Bisbey, Ph.D. at the 7th Annual Conference on Metapsychology in 1993.*

In 1990, I wrote an essay entitled "A Psychologist Looks at Metapsychology", which many of you have seen. In that piece, I talked about my initial entry into this field, included some of my personal history, and outlined the crucial differences between standard psychological techniques and metapsychological ones. This talk is really the next step. At the time I wrote that essay, I was in a transition phase of a continuing journey. Having completed that transition, today I would like to talk about it and about the journey in general.

I have actually been making two journeys, as I see it. They are somewhat intertwined. The first is my personal journey through life. The second, laid against the backdrop of the first, is my journey as a clinical psychologist with my clients (or viewers) through the process of therapy (facilitation). You will notice that I am using both the psychology and Metapsychology terms here. That is because I am going to speak from both frameworks. So please indulge me.

I want to begin where I left off in the essay I wrote during the transition. At that time, I was approaching completion of my training in Metapsychology in England. I had finished the General Facilitator Course and was just beginning the Technical Director training while concurrently doing an internship.

At that time, I was thinking in terms of both psychology theory and Metapsychology theory. By this, I mean simply that when I first saw a client or viewer, I found myself conceptualizing the case in both ways. I was still focusing on the similarities and differences between the two.

A case in point: my views concerning diagnosis. Though I have always firmly believed that labeling people is wrong, and that labeling the condition too often becomes labeling the person, my prior training in clinical psychology emphasized the value and utility of diagnosis—particularly in determining treatment planning. Consequently, when I started working with viewers, I still fit them into certain diagnostic categories. In so doing, I was indeed labeling the person rather than the condition. How, you may ask, did this happen, given the fact that my convictions about not labeling people were so strong? Habit is one answer I can give, but it's not a very satisfactory one. The actual change in thinking began when I was looking at the metapsychological concept of "having"—a concept that remains undefined in standard psychology.

## Having vs. Being

In his book Beyond Psychology, Dr. Gerbode talks about the ability to have as a basic ability that all people possess to varying degrees. He defines "having" as "the ability to be causative (or to act) with respect to an entity." He defines "entity" as "an object, event or relationship (state of affairs) that is part of a person's world, i.e. which exists, for a person, at a certain moment". He talks about the two ways in which we use the term "to have".

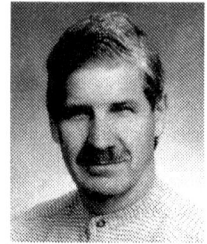

*Frank A. Gerbode,*
*M.D.*

The first is in referring to things external to our current identity; thus, for example, "I have a blue suit." The second is in referring to things internal or connected with our current identity; thus, "I have a bad temper." It was recognizing the confusion between these two usages that really changed my thinking about diagnosis.

I thought a lot about the ways in which we use—and confuse—the concepts of being and having. We often think of people in terms of their identities. For example, I might consider that John, a friend, "is intelligent". Very few people would be offended by such a statement. However, a better way of putting it would be to say "John has a high IQ." or "John has intelligence." The distinction may seem subtle, but it is important. "John has a high I.Q." or "John has intelligence" is a better way of expressing it, because although John's current identity may include being very intelligent, John as a person—his core identity—cannot be described solely with the statement that he is intelligent. And John can "step back from" his current identity—that "package" of qualities that he is "being" at the moment—and see the quality of intelligence as something he has (and therefore as something he can do something about), rather than thinking that it's just the way he is.

The distinction becomes clearer if we use a negative trait to describe the person. For example, if we were to say "John has a mental illness," we imply something quite different from what we imply in stating that "John is mentally ill." In the first in stance, we are describing the condition John has as something distinctly separate from himself or his core identity. In the second, we are describing John's core identity—who he fundamentally is—as being mentally ill.

Again, while this may seem to be a subtle distinction, it is actually powerful and important. When we say someone is something, we imply that the characteristic cannot be changed. We view—and suggest that others view—this characteristic as something inherent in the person's core identity. Whereas, when we say someone has something, we are implying that the characteristic can be changed because it is external to the being's core identity. We imply that it is one facet or possession, rather than a description of the whole.

It is important to note that in talking about what people have, I do not wish to validate the popular psychology idea of "having a disease". In recent years, it has become fashionable to say that people have the disease of alcoholism—meaning that alcoholism is a characteristic of them. The problem I have with this is that usually it is given as a reason for the person's being unable to change his condition; it gives responsibility and causation away. In labeling the condition a physical one that is simply part of the person and that therefore has no cure, we imply that there is nothing that can be done to change it.

People at Alcoholics Anonymous meetings state, "My name is _____ and I am an alcoholic." Alcoholism is thus seen as an integral as well as unalterable part of the person. While I am the first to admit that substance abuse is one of the most difficult areas to treat, I am not willing to assign those that abuse alcohol a label that implies that their behavior and resultant condition can never successfully be altered.

As psychiatrists or psychologists, we commonly refer to someone by his diagnosis: "Shirley is anorexic (or an anorexic)," or "Charlie is a psychopath." Such statements, although meant solely to describe a diagnosis or syndrome the person is exhibiting, in actuality end up constituting an overall description of the person, and one which is very limiting. They also imply that the person cannot change. Once someone has been diagnosed as having schizophrenia, he becomes "a schizophrenic" and retains that label for the rest of his life. If we look at Dr. Gerbode's definition of having, when we say someone has a condition, we are implying that it is something he can be causative over and therefore something that he can change.

In order to have a condition, character trait, or personality trait, one must have access to it and influence on it-and therefore have the ability to be causative or to act causatively with respect to it. Conceptually, this may be a bit more difficult to grasp than the idea of simple ownership—of having a car, or having a house. But take the example of "having a relationship" with another person. In order to have a relationship, one must have access to the other person (be able to perceive him, understand him, receive communication from him) and to have influence on the other person (be able to communicate to him, do things with him, act on him, etc.) One could not reasonably be said to have a relationship with another person with no interaction ever occurring between the two people. Take another example: having a condition like schizophrenia. In order to have schizophrenia—in the sense that I now use the word one would have to have access to the condition (experiencing its symptoms) and, potentially, one would be able to influence the condition. One could change it.

The degree to which we "have" corresponds to the degree to which we believe we embody access or influence on the object, person, perception, characteristic, phenomenon or condition. Often, people determine how happy are or how well they are doing in life by what they have, in terms both of material objects and of non-material phenomena—autos and anxieties, pools and paranoia, savings and symptoms. This explains how a person who appears to "have everything" can feel that he in fact "has nothing".

John has a house, a wife, a car, a child, a dog, money, a job, his health, an attractive appearance, his youth... as well as anxiety and depression. A friend "points out" that he "really" has nothing to be depressed about because he "has everything". But from John's viewpoint, he has nothing because he has problems with his house, he has little access to and influence on his wife (they do not communicate well), he has little access to and influence on his child (the child spends most of her time with his wife), he is bored at his job (he has mastered it and has no new goal), he doesn't consider his health to be something he has any control over, and he considers his youth and looks to be transitory and a result of happenstance and so has no causation over or influence on them,

And has anxiety—access to the symptoms, but no feeling he has influence over them.

And he has depression—access to the symptoms but, again, no feeling that he can influence them in any way.

John is unhappy.

Conversely, someone who looks as though he "has nothing" can in fact feel he "has everything". Jeff has no house, no job, little money and few possessions, fair health, his looks (such as they are), plans, and goals. From his viewpoint, he has what he needs. In his own estimation, he is adequately housed, able to find work, and he perceives himself as having access to and the ability to influence his health and his looks, as well as access to and the ability to affect his plans and goals. He feels, in short, that he has what he presently needs and wishes.

Jeff is happy.

The amount a person has of both external and internal phenomena—are central issues in how productive, satisfied, and happy he is in his current life. This area is frequently addressed in facilitation. In fact, when a person has successfully rid himself of a lot of charge, negative habits and behavior patterns, he often will experience a drop in "having"—a feeling of loss—simply because he has reduced the quantity of phenomena that he has access to and influence on, and has reduced the ways in which he has the past been causative in relation to himself and other people.

When a person considers himself to have less than what he requires or desires internally, he will frequently attempt to "boost" what he does have by taking on negative conditions or substituting external phenomena for internal ones. The person who eats sweets because she feels blue and doesn't have enough love or emotional nourishment is such a one, as is the person who drinks excessively because she doesn't have enough pleasant or relaxed feelings.

When I came to fully understand this concept of having, I stopped thinking in terms of diagnosis. The fact that a viewer had a diagnosable condition didn't lead to any kind of treatment plan and really added no extra information about a case (unless I was trying to get insurance reimbursement). Eventually, I could no longer find any valid reasons to think in terms of diagnosis. Instead, I began to think in terms of facilitation techniques to handle what the viewer presented to me. At this point, the only time I think in terms of diagnosis is when I have a viewer that may have a condition that makes facilitation difficult or impossible. This is a rare occasion.

Anyway, back to my journey. Somewhere during my Technical Director training and my internships following it, the theoretical underpinnings and basic assumptions of Metapsychology really became integrated. I was still at the stage where, upon meeting a client for the first time, I had a choice as to how to handle him. I could use the techniques of standard psychology or of Metapsychology, but I no longer felt I could mix the two effectively.

When did that happen? I'm not really sure. But somewhere along the way, I realized that the basic Rules of Facilitation (see http://www.tir.org/metapsy/rules.htm) were not only better but really necessary for long term resolution of psychological issues in therapy. That may sound like a pretty strong statement to make. It is.

## Interpreting for the Client

I came to this conclusion by looking at what happens in therapy and in life when I or anyone else violates them. One of the Rules states, in essence, "Thou shalt not interpret for the client." I started with that one -- fairly easy for me, because interpretation had always seemed to me a most glaring error in therapeutic technique. I knew from personal experience—as both client and therapist that interpretations are often rejected by the client. I had discovered that the reasons for this were varied. One reason was the obvious—the interpretation offered is simply wrong. This one didn't require explanation. It is commonly assumed in psychoanalytic practice that if the client rejects the analyst's interpretation, it means that the analyst is "encountering resistance", or that the client is "in denial". There is no suggestion that the analyst could be wrong.

Another reason was less obvious—the interpretation is right, but the client "isn't ready to accept it". Translation: the client isn't yet aware or responsible enough to accept the interpretation. But even if the client were able to accept the interpretation, the fact that he himself isn't the originator of this piece of wisdom makes a big difference. In facilitation, viewers often come up with realizations that sound exactly like classic psychoanalytic interpretations: "It was a decision I made when I was being potty trained-that I somehow always had to be neat and perfect—that caused this!" The difference is that the viewer has realized this; he has not been fed it by the facilitator. And when you come to realize something yourself, you know it, and that allows you to resolve once and for all the issue that the realization relates to. Not surprisingly, it also creates a tremendous feeling of release and freedom.

I learned from experience that no matter what pearls of wisdom I imparted in a therapy session, they didn't have the positive impact that the client's own realizations had. Furthermore, I found—not as a therapist, but as a facilitator—that when I did nothing but acknowledge and direct the client's attention, the impact was even more profound. The viewer would sort it out for himself. As I have said before, this is empowering and helps the viewer to be more causative.

Another thing I learned from experience was that in standard therapy, it was often the things I said to which I didn't attach much importance—that I didn't think were particularly polished pearls of wisdom—that had the most impact on my client. Whatever it was that I said would simply "spark off" something for the client:… cause or enable him to inspect something new… to realize something all on his own. And upon reflection, I came to realize that such catalytic communications on my part were seldom if ever interpretations, judgments, or suggestions. Rather, they were simply questions or acknowledgements.

Most of this pondering and comparing and evaluating I did not do consciously. It came to me in the form of realizations as I found myself using the Metapsychology techniques more and more ... and the tools of standard psychology less and less. At this time, I frequently asked my clients at the end of a program of facilitation or a course of therapy what they felt they had gained from the treatment. Consistently, viewers reported having resolved issues "once and for all", knowing with certainty the issues would not come back to haunt them. Many of my viewers tested this out by deliberately putting themselves in situations that would have triggered a lot of stuff in the past or by deciding to handle people with whom they had consistently had difficulty—much as we are wont, with some trepidation, to explore a broken and previously painful and sensitive tooth with our tongue after the dentist has repaired it. Routinely, they reported to me that they had been successful. The joy on their faces is indescribable.

Viewers who had been involved in therapy in the past had some comments to make that I feel are particularly relevant. Certainly they reinforced my enthusiasm for using metapsychological techniques as opposed to others. In the words of one viewer: "This is the first time in my life someone has listened to my story without interrupting me and without judging me in any way." And from another: "You didn't tell me what to find when I looked around, or what it meant. You helped me find my own meanings and I learned how to let go."

## "Letting Go"

"Letting go" is an interesting concept to me. I have heard it used in two contexts in psychology and other helping professions. The first appears in some of the popular psychology and self-help arenas. This is where the devotee is giving a lecture and makes the statement, "You have to let go of your past and your negative feelings." or "You have to let go and be yourself." A related context is the quasi-religious one, "Let go of this negativity. Let God (or whomever) take it away."

The second context is in more standard therapy methods where "letting go" is linked to "working through". A client "works through" something so he can "let go of it". The problem I have always had with all uses of the term "letting go" was that no one could ever tell me how to do it! No one had the slightest due how to teach someone to "let go", let alone how to "let go and be yourself". There was no program to let go, no definition of what letting go felt like, no point at which you knew you had let go. I found this all terribly frustrating as both a client and a clinician. The problem was that the basic idea itself felt right to me. The idea that in order to be happy and productive in the present one had to let go of the past made sense to me. I just couldn't figure out how to do it... or how to help someone else do it.

## "Working Through"

The standard therapy usage of this "working through" concept was even more frustrating. What does "working through" something actually mean? How do I help someone to work through something? It's a fuzzy term. When I asked people in the field, they usually said you work through by using interpretation, evaluation, or "unconditional positive regard", or they said it was "just the process of therapy". None of these were satisfactory answers, as far as I was concerned. I never felt comfortable with "working through" as a step in a treatment plan. In Mardi Horowitz' work on brief psychodynamic therapy for PTSD, this is the step that used to make me really angry. It's the step on the program that talks about "working through the issues" and "working through the transference issues". There is also the step that involves "working through resistances". He never says how one is supposed to do this. Nowhere in any of my graduate level psychology books, in fact, does one find a step by step guide to "working through" an issue with a client.

So, how does Metapsychology view the concepts of "working through" and "letting go"? I realized that in asking someone to view an area of concern repetitively—both by using techniques that are repetitive in nature and by using a variety of techniques sequentially to address a single area of concern -- I am indeed helping him to work through it. My new definition of "working through", then, is this: the process of inspecting an area from many different levels and angles until a realization or a number of realizations are produced that resolve that area. Following on that, "letting go" is simply what happens when a client has reached a major "end point" on an issue. The issue, whatever it was—a trauma, a failure in relationships, a painful inability—ceases to affect or concern the client.

A person has "let go" of something when he has inspected it to a point of resolution and it has ceased to be an ongoing issue in present time. It has become ... a part of the past. This is still a difficult concept to describe to new viewers and facilitators. The descriptions of an end point, while very thorough, still don't handle the fact that most people experientially don't understand what you are talking about. The best way to teach someone about end points is to enable him to experience one. Once he has done this, he can then give you examples from his past of other end points he has experienced.

The point that viewers usually make is that they knew they wouldn't be forced to leave a session without having handled something completely. They told me that I respected them enough to make sure they were all right before leaving a session. They also told me they felt they came prepared to work in session, despite the fact that they knew it might be painful. They felt able to confront the work because they knew they wouldn't feel terrible when they left the session. They pointed this out as a major difference between standard "50 minute hours" and the metapsychological approach—mandated by the Rules of Facilitation—of continuing to work until you reach an end point. Many viewers who had past therapy relate anecdotes of times they went to a therapy session and deliberately refrained from getting into whatever issue was upsetting them because they knew they would very likely become upset and leave feeling worse. They also speak of times where they were feeling too good to "get into" an issue in therapy because, again, they would get started and then have to leave feeling worse.

I realized recently [in 1993] that I am no longer able to tolerate a client's leaving a session before reaching an end point. Fortunately, using Metapsychology, I don't have to. Sometimes, however, circumstances prevent reaching a completely satisfactory end point. I never feel comfortable ending off when this occurs. I recently became aware of just how strongly I feel about this when I was offered the opportunity to do some work in another setting which would have required me to go back to using 50 minute hours. I realized that—given what I know now—I would feel I was being unethical were I to do this, and so turned down the opportunity. All of these observations are reflected in the Rules of Facilitation. When I recognized this, I realized I could no longer feel comfortable breaking these rules with a client.

Back to the journey… As it became easier for me to think with the theory behind Metapsychology techniques, I found I could design new techniques and programs to handle most of the situations my clients presented to me. Then I decided to take what was for me the ultimate step teaching others these techniques.

## Teaching Metapsychology

The first few that I taught were lay people, and so I had to learn how to explain the theory of Traumatic Incident Reduction (TIR) and Metapsychology in everyday terms. This was an extremely valuable experience. Like many professionals, I was largely unaware of how much jargon and sophisticated language I used when attempting to communicate to people on the subject of my profession. Through teaching lay people, I learned how to communicate concepts in English so that anyone who tried could understand them. This ability extended beyond explaining the theory of Metapsychology to explaining psychology and other related fields. The more I improved this ability, the better I was able to teach. I found that because I could explain in English, new viewers were better able to understand what they had to do when viewing. And because they understood the techniques better, the viewing went better as well.

It also allowed me to communicate the rationale behind what I do for a living without difficulty in ways that made sense to family and friends who are not in the field. When people asked me "What does therapy do?" or "Why do people go into therapy?" I could provide answers that made sense. In some cases, people who I thought would never be interested in any kind of growth or self-improvement became interested after I had given an explanation of the rationale behind TIR.

Then I began to teach people who had been trained in standard psychological methods—psychologists and counselors. This required me to think in terms of both theories again. Interestingly enough, I now find myself thinking in Metapsychological terms first and then translating back into psychological terms, rather than the reverse.

In 1992, when I was teaching a workshop on TIR to a group of counselors, I realized how thoroughly I had made the transition from psychology to Metapsychology. A student asked me if I judged clients out of session or predicted—out of session, to myself or others—what I would find with a given client in session. I actually had to think about this, and I realized that in fact I don't. I don't find myself thinking about a viewer's session data out of session except as it relates to case planning and technical direction—i.e. where do we go from here? I don't look at a viewer, in or out of session, and think about her issues. In session, my attention is on the viewer; I am not thinking about anything else. Out of session, if I am with a viewer, my attention is on her as a person, or on the subject of the conversation we are having and not on her issues or problems. I can have—and allow others to have—many identities apart from "issues".

How did this happen? I think it goes back to the larger journey, the backdrop onto which this secondary journey is laid. Because my experiences as a viewer have allowed me to handle a major portion of my own past issues and problems, these don't get triggered when I am working with others or in most social situations. I view the process of facilitation as a journey that parallels the journey of a person through life. I am helping people along this journey. My work with them as a facilitator represents only one small portion of their journey. That viewpoint allows me to see and appreciate the whole person instead of just the part of the person that is unhappy and in pain.

As a psychologist, this gives me much more freedom. I know I can help people. When I came across a problem as a technical director while drawing up a program for a viewer, I know I can adapt techniques to solve the problem, or ask someone else for input, and so ensure that my session agenda is in place well before I go into session with the viewer. I know that in my work, people get better. They get lasting results, and my certainty of that gives me the courage to try new things and the strength to stick by someone when things are tough. Though I know that I have limitations and that current Metapsychology theory has limitations, this isn't a problem for me. If I can't handle something, I refer to someone who can and in the meantime I try to come up with a way to expand the theory and techniques to address these things by communicating with other fully trained colleagues.

In Metapsychology, I have finally found a solid theoretical base that is nonetheless capable of expansion and change, and which lends itself to the development of new applications. This is very exciting for me. I have discovered that when I apply to a given area of psychological difficulty the basic concepts and principles of metapsychological theory—the Rules of Facilitation, the principles of effective communication, the concepts of having, of time and attention, of repetition, and so on—I can expand upon the theory and build new applications. As far as I am concerned, this is the true value of a good theory.

## Testing Metapsychology

A second mark of a good theory is its testability. Though research has its limitations because of the limitations of measurement instruments and in generalization from one subject group to another, it has value nonetheless. In my view it is essential to be able to show that various techniques do produce measurable changes. I suppose part of the reason I feel this way is that the field of academic psychology relies on research. Despite the fact of its never having been proven to work, psychodynamically oriented therapy is still in very common usage. This is because it hasn't been disproved either.

If you ask a client who has been undergoing psychoanalytic treatment for a few years what kinds of improvements he has experienced, he will probably reply with general statements and "feeling based" statements, and no specific statements of change. If you ask a viewer who has had some kind of facilitation what kinds of improvements he has experienced, he will probably reply with some general statements but he will also be able to give you specific statements of change— feelings have changed, behaviors have changed. I am not invalidating the gains an analysand may have experienced. However, I believe that people initially go into therapy not because they are seeking growth, but because they wish to relieve pain and to resolve difficulties. I don't feel today as if I have done my job correctly if a client leaves me without having thoroughly resolved at least most of the difficulties he came into viewing to address. The desire for growth is a good reason to continue in any kind of viewing activity. In my experience, though, it is not usually sufficient motivation to start any kind of viewing activity. This doesn't mean I will turn away a viewer who comes into viewing for self-growth. What I mean is that people rarely seek out my help for growth alone. There is almost always some area in their lives they are unhappy with that has prompted them to see a therapist or to do some viewing.

So the fact that we can test these theories and techniques is very appealing to me. My doctoral dissertation is a treatment outcome study comparing TIR, another treatment, and a control group for outcome with crime victims who have Post-Traumatic Stress Disorder. However as well as advocating that we undertake controlled treatment outcome studies on Metapsychological techniques, I would like to recommend that practitioners start collecting data for single subject design studies routinely. Single case studies are a valid method of testing a treatment technique. They are not very difficult to design or interpret, requiring merely that one get together some good instruments and ask new clients to complete them—pre-viewing, post-viewing, and ideally again at a point perhaps six months after they have completed viewing.. If you do enough of them, they add a lot of new information to the field. I think this would be a very valuable project to undertake for those of us using Metapsychology techniques. I feel a responsibility to discover and prove what works with whom and if possible why. This information helps me to be a better technical director and also helps me to decide what to use and what not to use in the future.

Using this theory and these techniques has other benefits for me. At the end of a long day of facilitation, I don't feel drained as I often did when I was using other techniques. Most of the time I know I have accomplished something, so I don't feel frustrated as I used to be in the past. When I am upset about a case or having difficulty handling an issue, I speak to my technical director and come up with a new approach. If an issue of mine has been triggered, I have a session.

In fact though I may feel tired at the end of a long day, I often feel in quite high spirits as well. Being able to watch someone go from confusion to certainty, from sadness to happiness in a single session is a wonderful privilege. It is invigorating. I get the same satisfaction and joy from teaching Metapsychology techniques to others. I value my students and their contributions. I have not yet taught a workshop or a course in which I did not learn something from my students. Their questions force me to examine the theory more closely and often provoke realizations about my own engagement with the theory and techniques. It's also very exciting to watch my students make some of the discoveries I have made over the last few years about the utility of the theory and its techniques. I enjoy their enthusiasm and commitment.

Both my journeys go on and my enthusiasm for the theory and techniques of Metapsychology continues unabated. The more I do, the more useful I find the pursuit. I would like to acknowledge those of you who have played a part in helping me to find this new way of viewing people, the world, and the helping professions. Thank you.

# Brief Treatment of Trauma–Related Symptoms In Incarcerated Females with TIR

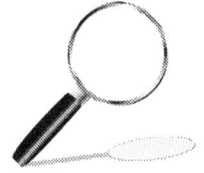

**3**

## By Pamela Vest Valentine, Ph.D.

Pamela V. Valentine is an Assistant Professor in the Social Work Program at the School of Social and Behavioral Sciences at the University of Alabama. Dr. Valentine obtained her Ph.D. from Florida State University in 1997. The following article is based on materials presented at the *Proceedings of the Tenth National Symposium on Doctoral Research in Social Work* (1998).

## Statement of the Research Problem

Conducted in the Tallahassee Federal Correction Institute (FCI) in Florida, this experimental outcome study examined the effectiveness of Traumatic Incident Reduction (TIR) (Gerbode, 1989) in treating trauma-related symptoms of female inmates who were victims of interpersonal violence. TIR is a brief (in this case, one session), straightforward, memory-based, therapeutic intervention most similar to imaginal flooding. A memory-based intervention implies that the symptoms currently experienced by a client are related to a past event and that lasting resolution of those symptoms involves focusing on the memory rather than focusing on symptom management. TIR is straightforward in that the roles of both the client and therapist are very clearly defined and strictly followed.

TIR is both a client-respectful and therapist-directed intervention. It is client-respectful in that the client's perception of the traumatic incident takes precedence over the therapist's perception of the incident. For example, should the client have multiple traumatic events in her past, she would choose the event to focus on during the one-session TIR intervention, and her version of the event would be undisputed by the therapist. Additionally, an event is considered traumatic if the client so deems it. In other words, the client, not the therapist, is considered the expert regarding the client's life and the impact of the traumatic event on her life. TIR is a therapist-directed technique in that the therapist acts as a guide, not an interpreter, evaluator or problem solver. Both the non-intrusive stance of the therapist and the client's work of confronting the painful incident combine to empower the client (Valentine & Smith, 1996).

The study specifically examined the effectiveness of TIR on symptoms of posttraumatic stress disorder (PTSD), depression, anxiety, and low expectancy of success (i.e., low self-efficacy). Symptoms of PTSD include intrusion, avoidance, and arousal (American Psychological Association, 1994; Waldinger, 1990). Intrusion involves nightmares, recurring thoughts and flashbacks. Avoidance speaks of numbing of feelings, avoiding places associated with the event, and attempts to refrain from thinking about the event. Arousal, among other things, pertains to an exaggerated startle response and hypervigilance. The diagnosis of PTSD means that the symptoms are more present after the traumatic event than they were before the event, and that the symptoms have existed for at least four weeks. Other symptoms associated with trauma are low self-esteem and a reduced sense of being in control.

The theoretical underpinnings of TIR are considerable and are closely related to the etiology of trauma-related symptoms. Psychodynamic theorists explain the effects of trauma as consequences of unresolved emotional processing that occurred during a traumatic episode (Gerbode, 1989). Behaviorists write of classical conditioning and seek treatment that reveals the stimuli associated with a particular traumatic event (Resnick, Kilpatrick, & Lipovsky, 1991). Cognitive theorists speculate that one's basic beliefs about the world were shattered during the traumatic event and that the shattered beliefs cry out to be restored (Janoff-Bulman, 1992). Cathartic theory, on which TIR is primarily based, agrees with each of the above conceptualizations. It also asserts that a heightened physiological state (much like the state experienced in the original incident) must be recreated to finish the emotional processing and to reveal the associated stimuli and/or the distorted cognitive schema (Straton, 1990). TIR is structured so that the incident is viewed repetitively, non-intrusively, and in an open-ended time frame. The activity is designed to elicit a heightened physiological state so that the client can process the event to its completion (Gerbode, 1989). The open-ended time frame is crucial in allowing the client to emotionally engage in the memory without fear of being cut off.

There are several reasons for studying the influence of TIR on previously traumatized female inmates. Since 1980, the rate of family homicide has increased fivefold (Joffe, Wilson, & Wolfe, 1986). Women are the target of much violence, as illustrated by the following: 75% of adult women have been victims of at least one sexual assault, robbery, or burglary (Resnick, et al., 1991); and 53.7% are victims of more than one crime. Abundant data suggest that PTSD can result from having been a victim of crime or having witnessed a violent crime (Astin, Lawrence, & Foy, 1993; Breslau, Davis, Andreski & Peterson, 1991; Resnick, et al., 1991). Therefore, the number of women affected by PTSD is growing as violence and sexual abuse increase in society as a whole (Ursano & Fullerton, 1990). There is a lack of empirical research on the traumatic effects of interpersonal violence (e.g. robbery, rape, incest, physical assault). Since inmates are typically victims of interpersonal violence (Gabel, Johnston, Baker, & Cannon, 1993), the inmate population studied was particularly suitable for TIR.

Another reason for studying the influence of TIR on previously traumatized female inmates is the increased number of female prisoners in the last decade (Gabel, et al., 1993; "As Inmates Pay, so do Kids," 1995). This increase is due to a boost in drug-related arrests and sentencing. Between 1980 and 1989, 25% of women in police custody were arrested for buying drugs; whereas among men, drug purchases accounted for only 10% of the arrests. More arrested females regularly use drugs than do their male counterparts.

Among women incarcerated for violent crimes, a 1991 study (US Department of Justice, 1991) found that 61% of female inmates had victimized a male and that 36% had close relationships with their victims (Gabel, et al., 1993). Violent offenders with a history of physical or sexual abuse are more likely to have killed relatives or intimates than strangers. In contrast, female inmates with no prior history of abuse were more likely to have victimized a stranger while committing a robbery. These statistics suggest a connection between female victimization and women who victimize. The impact of unresolved trauma needs to be explored.

The traditional treatment of inmates seldom incorporates the influence of prior traumatic events on current behavior (A. McNeece, personal communication, 4/18/1995). Furthermore, most trauma treatment is lengthy and nonspecific, making it difficult to reach conclusions about treatment efficacy. The above reasons mandated the need for this study.

Finally, while both clients and therapists throughout the United States report that TIR alleviates trauma-related symptoms (Valentine & Smith, 1996), little experimental research has been conducted to substantiate such claims (see next section). By conducting an experimental outcome study on the effects of TIR on traumatized, female inmates, knowledge is built pertaining to (1) the effectiveness of TIR, and to (2) the treatment of victims of interpersonal violence.

## Prior Research on TIR

Although advocates of TIR suggest that it is a highly effective and cost-efficient brief treatment modality, there is little research to justify such claims. Most of what is written about TIR is anecdotal. A case study (Valentine, 1995), a multisite clinical debriefing study (Valentine & Smith, 1998), a dissertation based on a quasi-experimental design (Coughlin, 1995), and another dissertation, a true experimental study based on victims of crime in England (Bisbey, 1995), comprise the body of TIR studies.

The studies by Valentine (1995) and Valentine and Smith (1998) used ethnographic methods and were qualitative and discovery oriented. The client perspectives gathered in these studies expanded and clarified the existing theory base of TIR. The former study provided a vivid case study of the application of TIR in an outpatient setting. The latter study employed extensive phone interviews of the experiences of four clients living in three states who were treated by three certified TIR practitioners. Although the research designers did not allow conclusions about the efficacy of the intervention protocol, clients' and clinicians' enthusiasm about their experiences led the authors to conduct a controlled clinical trial of TIR.

The current study employed a credible design with a three-month follow-up and relied on multiple published measures of anxiety, depression, PTSD and general satisfaction. Furthermore, the sample consisted of female inmates who represented different ethnic groups and diverse socioeconomic classes. Finally, it used an analytic strategy that allowed conclusions about whether the treatment and control conditions differed after treatment and at a follow-up interval. Although the study was not intended to be a definitive test of TIR, it provides a rigorous examination of its efficacy with women of color from varied socioeconomic classes.

## Research Questions

This study addressed the following research questions:

1. How does TIR influence PTSD-related symptoms in incarcerated females?
2. How does TIR influence intrusion?
3. How does TIR influence avoidance?
4. How does TIR influence arousal?
5. How does TIR influence anxiety?
6. How does TIR influence depression?
7. How does TIR influence sense of control?

## Methodology—Clients

Subjects in the study were recruited from the Federal Correction institute (FCI), Tallahassee, Florida. The sample was drawn from the total number of inmates at the facility (N = 730). The population (N = 730) filled out a Participation Questionnaire to indicate interest in the study. This questionnaire was used to determine eligibility based on whether inmates (1) had experienced a prior trauma in their lives, and if so, the nature of the trauma; (2) had experienced one or more of the trauma-related symptoms; and (3) were willing to further discuss their traumatic experience with a mental health professional. 248 inmates met the initial criteria. The inmates were brought together, in groups of approximately 12, to have the study explained to them and to have them sign consent forms when they chose to participate. 148 agreed to take part and were randomly assigned to either treatment or control conditions. 25 subsequently withdrew from the study, leaving 123 subjects. The reasons for withdrawal varied and included work-assignment constraints, disinterest, self-reevaluation of their level of traumatization, and/or a change of heart.

Average age of inmates in the treatment condition was 32.8 years (SD = 9.1), and the average age of those in the control condition was 34.9 (SD = 9.8). The majority of the participants were Black (50%), 38.5% were White, and 24% identified themselves as Hispanic. 32% of participants had never been married, and the treatment and control conditions did not differ significantly on marital status. 35% of the participants had no high school diploma whereas another 35% had some college or vocational training. The treatment and control conditions did not different significantly among age, racial distribution, marital status or educational level.

The following exclusion criteria were used: inmates who were on antipsychotic medication; inmates who had been hospitalized within the last three years with a diagnosis of bipolar disorder or schizophrenic disorder; inmates experiencing a severe depressive episode that required immediate psychiatric hospitalization; inmates experiencing hallucinations, delusions, or bizarre behavior; inmates with an alcohol or drug abuse disorder; or inmates who were victimized within three months prior to participation in the study. These criteria were in part modeled after the Foa study (Foa, Rothbaum, Riggs, & Murdock, 1991) and the recommendations of clinicians in the correctional facility. In general, the exclusion criteria represented acute situations that would be counterproductive to the process of TIR.

## Methodology—Practitioners

All TIR practitioners were female; had graduate degrees in social work, marital and family therapy, or psychology. They had a mean age of thirty-five, with 7.2 years clinical experience on average. They were given sixteen hours of training in TIR by a certified TIR instructor. Practitioners delivered TIR using a standardized protocol in three to four hour blocks to every client in the treatment condition. A comprehensive treatment manual was created in order to control for differing practitioner skills. Random sessions were audiotaped, and an independent observer who was well versed in the TIR protocol reviewed sections of the tapes to ensure treatment integrity. Alpha was set a .05, beta was set at .20 , and the effect size was estimated at .50.

The primary hypothesis of the study follows: Those inmates receiving TIR will experience significant reduction in one or more of their self-reported PTSD-related symptoms, while those in the control conditions will not.

While all subjects completed pretest, posttest, and follow-up tests, additional steps were required of those in the experimental condition. Those steps were: (1) have a one-on-one orientation to learn the nature of TIR and the roles that the inmates and the mental health practitioners would play, (2) receiving a session of TIR, and (3) completing a debriefing session.

## Results

The instruments used to determine the efficacy of TIR on trauma-related symptoms were the PTSD Symptom Scale (PSS), the Beck Depression Inventory (BDI), the Clinical Anxiety Scale (CAS) and the Generalized Expectancy of Success Scale (GESS). These instruments were administered in a pretest, posttest, and three-month follow-up format.

To analyze the data, an ANCOVA (with the pretest as the covariate) was conducted on each of the above measures, as well as on the three subscales of the PSS: intrusion, avoidance, and hyper-arousal. Analysis revealed that TIR showed significant differences at the .05 level on the PSS, the BDI, the CASE, and the GESS at both posttest and the three-month follow-up. In other words, both times, the experimental condition showed a statistically significant *decrease* in symptoms of posttraumatic stress disorder (and its related subscales) and of depression and anxiety, while those in the control condition remained approximately the same. Subjects assigned to the experimental condition *improved* on the measure of self-efficacy at a statistically significant level, while subjects assigned to the control condition did not. The null hypothesis was rejected, and the research hypothesis confirmed.

Although the results of this study were promising, care should be taken in generalizing to larger populations. For example, while we demonstrated TIR's effectiveness in treating trauma-related symptoms in female inmates, it would be a mistake to assume that TIR is effective with male inmates, or with female inmates in different institutional settings, or with persons outside a prison setting. Additional studies should be undertaken with those populations before definitive conclusions are drawn about TIR's more general efficacy. Besides testing TIR's effectiveness on different populations, TIR should be compared against other brief trauma treatments. Finally, research implications involve testing TIR's effectiveness on different ethnic groups and discovering the variables associated with training therapists to deliver TIR to a variety of ethnic groups.

## Implications for Social Work Practice

The implications for social work practice are multiple. Social work's knowledge base is increased in realizing an effective trauma intervention with female inmates. The knowledge base would be increased further by researching (1) TIR's effectiveness with other populations; (2) TIR as compared with other brief trauma interventions; (3) and the implementation of TIR with various ethnic groups.

One primary practice implication pertains to the accessibility of TIR to social workers in a variety of settings. TIR is an unfranchised therapeutic intervention. While social workers should be trained to deal with clients' traumatic memories, Gerbode (1989), the originator of TIR, does not require licensure nor certification to practice TIR, making TIR more accessible to a greater number of social workers. Furthermore, TIR training usually costs a fraction of the price of other trauma-focused interventions. Social work educators continually search for effective practice modalities that can be taught to students. Because TIR follows a detailed treatment protocol, it represents a practice model that can be easily taught to students within schools of social work. [Ed. Note: TIR Workshop attendees can now receive Continuing Education units approved by the National Association of Social Workers].

From a practice perspective, it is also noteworthy that addressing only one item from the list of traumatic events still brought about statistically and clinically significant results in the inmates. This underscores that assessing for traumatic events will not necessarily embroil practitioners in very lengthy treatment procedures. Instead, the results suggest that substantive issues can be addressed in only one session. Such results define a win-win situation for both clients and practitioners.

The comments given by inmates suggest that they were highly appreciative of the client-respectful nature of TIR. For many of them, this was their first experience with a treatment provider who was both effective and respectful. Given the histories of victimization cited by inmates, this feature represents one of the most important contributions of this intervention protocol.

Another practice implication is the applicability of this technique to the population of social workers' typical clients. Many clients are oppressed and have likely been traumatized; yet, few psychosocial interview protocols exist that focus on the effects of trauma. Therefore, the demonstration of the effectiveness of TIR with previously traumatized female inmates should have several practice implications: (1) inclusion of a history of prior traumatic events in assessment of client problems; (2) inclusion of prior traumatic events in the treatment plan designed for the client; (3) encouragement of social workers to be trained to administer brief treatment to traumatized clients; and (4) practice of TIR by agency-based social workers, understanding that TIR has demonstrated effectiveness against trauma-related symptoms in incarcerated females. This study has shown TIR to be effective in the treatment of traumatized federally incarcerated females and renders TIR a promising intervention that begs further research.

# References

American Psychiatric Association, (1994), *Diagnostic and Statistical Manual of Mental Disorders* (4th Ed.). Washington, DC; author.

"As Inmates Pay, so do Kids: More Mothers Jailed, Researchers Say." (1995 May). *NASW News.* 40(5), 7.

Astin, M. Lawrence, K., Foy, D. (1993) Posttraumatic Stress Disorder Among Battered Women: Risk and Resiliency Factors. *Violence and Victims*, (8), 17-28.

Bisbey, L.B. (1995). *No longer a victim: a treatment outcome study of crime victims with post-traumatic stress disorder.* Doctoral dissertation for California School of Professional Psychology, San Diego. UMI publication number 9522269.

Breslau, Davis, Andreski & Peterson (1991) Traumatic events and posttraumatic stress disorder in an urban population of young adults. Arch Gen Psychiatry 48(3):216-222.

Coughlin, W.E. (1995). *Traumatic Incident Reduction: Efficacy in treating anxiety symptomatology.* UMI publication number 9537919.

Foa, Rothbaum, Riggs, & Murdock, (1991). Treatment of posttraumatic stress disorder in rape victims: A comparison between cognitive-behavioral procedures and counseling. *Journal of Consulting and Clinical Psychology, 59,* 715-723.

Gabel, K., Johnston, D., Baker, B., & Cameron, H. (1993) Female Offenders. Prepared for the *Encyclopedia of the National Association of Social Workers.*

Gerbode, F. (1989). *Beyond Psychology: An Introduction to Metapsychology.* Palo Alto: IRM Press.

Janoff-Bullman, B. (1992). *Shattered Assumptions.* New York: The Free Press.

Joffe, P., Wilson, S., & Wolfe, D. (1986). "Promoting Changes in Attitudes and Understanding of Conflict Resolution Among Child Witness of Family Violence." *Canadian Journal of Behavioural* Science, 18, 356-366.

Resnick, H.S., Kilpatrick, D.G., and Lipovsky, J.A. (1991) *Profile of Jail Inmates, 1989*. NDJ-9097. Washington, DC: Bureau of Justice Statistics.

Straton (1990). Catharsis reconsidered. Australian *and New Zealand Journal of Psychiatry*, 24, 543-551.

Ursano, R. & Fullerton, C. (1990). "Cognitive and Behavioral Responses to Trauma." Journal of Applied Psychology, 20 (21), 1766-1775.

Snell, Tracy L. and Morton, Danielle C. (1991), *Women in Prison, Survey of State Inmates*, Washington, DC: Bureau of Justice Statistics/

Valentine, P.V. (1995). "Traumatic Incident Reduction: A review of a new intervention." *Journal of Family Psychotherapy*, 6, (2), 79-85.

Valentine, P.V. & Smith, T.E. (1996, November). *Brief Treatment of Traumatized Clients: An Ethnographic Study*. Paper presented at the annual meeting of the National Association of Social Workers in Cleveland, OH.

Waldinger, R.J. (1990) *Psychiatry for Medical students*. (2nd Ed.). Washington, DC: American Psychiatric Press.

# 4 TIR and Anxiety Symptomatology

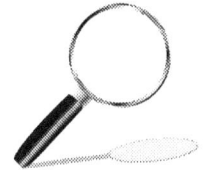

## By Wendy Coughlin, Ph.D.

No outcome evaluation studies of Traumatic Incident Reduction (TIR) had yet been done in 1992. Its efficacy had not been established except through anecdotal evidence offered by proponents of the methodology. As I began doctoral study, I was intent on finding tools to remove blocks to therapeutic progress. After attending a seminar introducing TIR, it became clear that Traumatic Incident Reduction worked to resolve these barriers. It seemed logical to develop a research project to evaluate its therapeutic utility. Only one other study had begun, a comparison of TIR and DTE (Direct Therapeutic Exposure) being conducted by Lori Beth Bisbey in England.

The premise for the study of TIR included several initial assumptions. First, it was clear that therapeutic barriers often occur when an individual attempts to avoid addressing sensitive material. Second, the sensitive material frequently has a traumatic content.[1] Third, the barrier needs to be resolved so that the individual can deal with the traumatic material. This allows the person to desensitize to it, and cognitively restructure its meaning so that it is no longer aversive material. Traumatic Incident Reduction satisfied the three major known components required to address therapeutic impasses.

In 1992, I lacked the resources for mounting a full-scale study. Anyone familiar with the requirements of outcome evaluation research can attest to the complexity of conducting a fully replicable investigation. There were few mental health clinicians certified to conduct TIR. No preliminary data was available to guide further research. And, the Institute for Research in Metapsychology (IRM) was anxious to publish data to substantiate the utility of the procedure. In order to bring supporting evidence to the professional community as quickly as possible, a pilot study was developed using a quasi-experimental pre-test/post-test design. Anxiety was chosen as the most clearly measurable component of both therapeutic avoidance and traumatic response. A subgroup of individuals with panic symptoms was also assessed.

Efficacy studies measure the impact of treatment. To best measure that impact in the most realistic setting available, the research was conducted in private practice settings of established facilitators of Traumatic Incident Reduction[2]. A list of qualified facilitators was provided by The Institute for Research in Metapsychology. TIR is a standardized procedure. Therefore, delivery of service does not vary among practitioners. This feature made it possible to compare the outcomes of service provided by different individuals. All participating facilitators signed an affidavit to attest to their adherence to the official TIR protocol. Due to the simplicity of the procedure, it is not necessary to have clinical background in order to administer it. TIR also includes ground rules

(See http://www.tir.org/metapsy/rules.htm), which generate both empathy and a safe therapeutic space. It not only does not require therapist insight, but it prohibits interference from, or customization by, the facilitator.

When taught and supervised by a certified TIR trainer, any adult with average intellect can execute the procedure. According to TIR developers Gerbode and French (1992):

> "We have found that *anyone* of good will and reasonable intelligence who wants to be able to help people who are unhappy can become a competent facilitator."

Although some of those providing data for this research did possess substantial mental health background, some did not. The initial experimental design had to be modified to accommodate facilitators who did not have a background in mental health.

Originally, we hoped to pre-select our study participants to include only those suffering from anxiety or panic disorders. This was only possible if there was an initial diagnosis, but not all participating facilitators were qualified to diagnose. Thus, we were not able to screen participants. In the end this proved more valuable than problematic. Our data indicate efficacy for a broad range of anxiety levels including those customarily experienced by normal people in normal environments. In short, because of this seeming limitation, the results are more validly applicable to a general population.

Two instruments were used to assess clients. A standardized and well validated test of anxiety, The State-Trait Anxiety Inventory (STAI) (Spielberger, 1983) was used to evaluate State and Trait Anxiety levels. State Anxiety represents immediate feelings of apprehension and tension, the anxiety a person feels "at the moment." Trait Anxiety reflects the individual's tendency to respond to the world in an anxious fashion. State Anxiety is generally amenable to short-term therapeutic interventions whereas Trait Anxiety tends to be an enduring characteristic of the individual. I specifically designed the second scale for this study. It was The Symptom Checklist, intended to elicit the symptoms of panic as defined by the diagnostic criteria set down in the DSM-IV (APA, 2000). Symptom checklists allow individuals to directly rate the presence or absence of specific symptoms. There is a high degree of reliability as they represent a direct report from the client and are free from researcher bias. Neither instrument required facilitator interpretation.

## Method

Six facilitators trained in TIR provided data from their private practice. A total of twenty-five participants commenced, but five withdrew for reasons not related to this study. Each participant completed both the STAI and The Symptom Checklist on three occasions: on intake, and on one and three month follow-ups. The efficacy of Traumatic Incident Reduction as a treatment tool for managing anxiety and panic was assessed by a change in the reported symptom levels before and after treatment.

## Results

There was a substantial and statistically significant reduction in State Anxiety for the entire sample. State Anxiety levels dropped by nearly one third of their original levels. Looking at the scoring on the STAI, the drop moved the group average from an anxiety level which would cause clinical concern and personal discomfort to a level that is considered normal for most people. The reduction in State Anxiety remained significant three months after treatment ended. Trait Anxiety levels also decreased by approximately twenty percent and held steady over the three month post-treatment period. These results indicate that Traumatic Incident Reduction is very effective in reducing anxiety. It is noteworthy that the reduction in anxiety levels occurred both for those in the normal pre-test range of anxiety as well as for those whose anxiety levels began at a higher, clinically significant level. This demonstrates that TIR is an effective tool for anyone. It will help those whose anxiety creates a problem in their life to bring that anxiety to tolerable levels. It will also help those who are only mildly anxious, perhaps only voicing reasonably normal concerns about their life, to reduce their discomfort and achieve a state of less worry and greater calm. Interestingly, there were no significant differences in the reduction of State or Trait Anxiety levels for individuals who also had panic disorder and those that did not suffer panic. There were, however, major differences in the level of panic symptoms. There were no additional follow-ups past three months.

Panic is defined as a discrete period of intense fear with symptoms of extreme anxiety such as pounding heart, shaking, shortness of breath, nausea, and fears of going crazy or dying [3]. Seven members of the study reported having at least one panic attack in the previous month. The average length of treatment time for the panic group was 10.3 hours with a range between 3 hours and 24 hours of treatment contact. In that relatively brief period, the mean number of panic attacks decreased from 12.1 to 1.1. That represents a 91% reduction in the number of panic attacks. Additionally, the number and severity of the symptoms decreased substantially. There was a 64% reduction in the number of usual symptoms. The number of severe symptoms decreased by 67%. For individuals who suffer from panic disorder, this results in a marked improvement in their quality of life. It is important to note that these results occurred without the need to use sedating, often addictive, medications which are commonly prescribed to manage panic disorder.

The sample group was subdivided, based on the presence or absence of panic and the levels of State and Trait Anxiety. The general trends and results were similar across groups with one important exception. The group that suffered from panic and had low State Anxiety scores reported an approximately 25% increase in State Anxiety and a 50% increase in Trait Anxiety following treatment.

Further research needs to be done to determine the cause of this aberrant response. One possible explanation relates to the function of the panic attack for some individuals. A panic attack may serve as a psychological mechanism to "hold" or release anxiety. Once the panic symptomatology has been dispersed, related anxieties manifest as both State and Trait anxiety symptoms. While this appears to be objectively problematic, it is subjectively more manageable. An individual with State or Trait Anxiety can manage those symptoms with cognitive behavioral tools. State and Trait anxiety are more amenable to control and management than panic. Any treatment intervention which returns conscious control to the individual is usually considered beneficial.

## Discussion

Traumatic Incident Reduction is an effective technique for reducing many types and symptoms of anxiety. The most debilitating presentation of anxiety is the panic attack. TIR is highly effective in reducing the number of panic attacks, the number of symptoms experienced during a panic attack and the severity of the symptoms. The procedure of viewing used in TIR allows the individual to revisit his/her panic symptoms and begin to understand why they occur. Once an understanding is present, the individual is able to take conscious control over the symptoms. The most frightening aspect of most panic attacks is that the individual does not know what is happening. Frequently, panic originates with an earlier, fearful event that has been forgotten by the individual. Because TIR does not proceed in a logical, linear fashion, it may unlock the memory and reveal the significance of panic symptoms more readily than traditional therapeutic approaches.

State Anxiety, which is nervousness about an event or situation, is highly responsive to treatment using TIR. One might normally encounter this type of anxiety prior to an important event, during public speaking or when making a major life change. Anxiety can be defined as "anticipatory fear". Based on past experience, we anticipate that the approaching event contains an element of danger. Traumatic Incident Reduction allows the individual to investigate the interconnecting cognitions which may link a past event with a current event and the belief that there is danger. In re-viewing the linked events, a clearer understanding may be achieved and, through cognitive rehearsal, the individual may come to feel less fear. In this way, TIR may facilitate the reduction in State Anxiety.

Once an individual begins to evaluate the origins of his/her anxiety, once he/she has gained control over overt symptoms, there is often an enhanced sense of competence in handling life. The reduction in Trait Anxiety may result from an overall sense of enhanced mastery that can be the outcome of using Traumatic Incident Reduction. Of those people who began with clinically significant levels of Trait Anxiety, 69% had this score reduced to within the normal range. "Cure" is often defined as eliminating the deviation from the norm. It can therefore be suggested that TIR cures pathological levels of Trait Anxiety approximately 70% of the time.

Figures and efficacy of this magnitude are seldom found in traditional psychotherapeutic modalities, given that the average length of treatment was 13 hours which would on average have occurred in only 4-5 sessions. It can be postulated that the extraordinary treatment outcome was related to practitioner expertise. However, this would not be a valid assumption. Facilitator expertise was determined only to assure adherence to the protocol. Treatment administration does not deviate from one provider to another among those fully trained to provide TIR. The language and response patterns are specifically scripted so as not to vary among presentations. Unlike most forms of psychotherapy, TIR does rely on practitioner talent to provide results. It requires only adherence to the protocol for administration.

## Comparisons to Other Modalities

The parsimony in explaining why Traumatic Incident Reduction works lies in its incorporation of knowledge gleaned from the main schools of psychotherapy.

Psychodynamic theories approach symptoms as signals of unconscious material. Freud identified anxiety as originating in events that threatened the individual. Psychodynamic therapy focuses on uncovering the originating incidents and releasing the unconscious material leading to enhanced understanding which typically causes the symptoms to decrease or disappear. Traumatic Incident Reduction addresses incidents in an individual's life which were 'traumatic'. When the impact of those incidents is 'reduced' the symptoms decrease or disappear.

Behavioral theories view anxiety as a conditioned response. Behavioral treatments therefore focus on extinguishing the conditioned response through desensitization. A behavioral protocol would require the individual to repeatedly be exposed to anxiety-inducing stimuli without reinforcing (responding to) the anxiety. After repeated exposure, the individual becomes desensitized and no longer responds with anxiety. Treating anxiety with Traumatic Incident Reduction similarly requires the repeated viewing of incidents related to the symptom, releasing affect until the individual no longer responds with the symptom.

Cognitive theorists view the underlying belief systems of the individual as the foundation to healthy or unhealthy responses to the world. Foa and Kozak (1985) view pathological anxiety as originating in previously stored "fear programs" contained in the informational network of the memory. To resolve symptoms, the therapist assists the clients in uncovering their "fear programs" in order to reevaluate their validity. Typically, once the symptom producing "program" is uncovered, it is recognized as containing irrational beliefs. Once identified, the irrational beliefs can be reframed thus eliminating the symptom. Thematic TIR asks the viewer to identify "an incident that could have caused" the symptom and to chain back through events connected to the symptom. Once the salient events are re-viewed, the viewer is able to determine possibly erroneous decisions that were made at the time of the incident and re-evaluate their validity. Once that material is identified, the viewer is free to reframe the incident and resolve the symptom(s) connected to it.

The essential difference between traditional treatment modalities and Traumatic Incident Reduction lies in the role of the practitioner. Traditional treatments evolving from psychological theories rely on a therapist to conduct and interpret the treatment. TIR relies only on an individual to facilitate the procedure. The full implication of this difference is beyond the scope of this chapter. However, several benefits are clear: TIR does not require years of collegiate study to prequalify the provision of assistance to others. The efficacy of TIR is not contingent on the unique talents of a particular facilitator. The procedure is standardized and does not require continuous adjustments. It is universally applicable to anyone of average intellect who is able to focus sufficiently to follow the procedure. Most importantly, Traumatic Incident Reduction does not allow interference from the practitioner. I believe that it is precisely the prohibition against interpretation and discussion that frees the individual to investigate his/her cognitive content in order to uncover the specific cause of his/her specific symptoms without bias. This freedom allows for the efficient and precise resolution of symptoms using Traumatic Incident Reduction.

## End Notes

[1] The term "trauma" is used herein in the broadest sense of the term. Material is traumatic when it threatens the physical or psychological life of the individual.

[2] At the time The Institute for Research in Metapsychology, headed by Frank A. Gerbode, the developer of TIR, credentialed all research facilitators.

[3] For a full definition of panic disorder consult The Diagnostic and Statistical Manual of Mental Disorders (4th edition).

## References

American Psychiatric Association (2000). *Diagnostic and Statistical Manual of Mental Disorders*, 4<sup>th</sup> ed. Washington, DC: Author.

Foa, E.B. & Kozak, M.J. (1985) Treatment of anxiety disorders: Implications for psychopathology. In A.H. Tuma & J.D. Maser (Eds.) *Anxiety and Anxiety Disorders* (pp. 421-461). Hillsdale, NJ: Lawrence Erlbaum.

French, G.D. & Gerbode, F.A. (1992). *The Traumatic Incident Reduction Workshop*. Menlo Park, CA: IRM Press.

Spielberger, C. D. (1983). *Manual for the State-Trait Anxiety Inventory (STAI)*. PaloAlto, CA: Consulting Psychologists Press.

# 5 Trauma Resolution in an At-Risk Youth Program

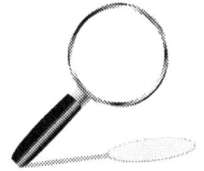

## By Teresa Descilo, MSW, CTS

From 2001 to 2003, Victim Services Center of Miami received funding from the Department of Juvenile Justice in Florida to help at-risk youth resolve the impact of trauma. At-risk youth were defined as children who had risk factors in three of four domains—school, family, substance abuse and behavior. We primarily provided services at Madison Middle School, an inner city school in the Miami area zip code with the highest juvenile crime rate. Madison hosts approximately 1300 students from grades 6 to 8. In a recent year, 20.7% of the students missed more than a month of school per year. Compared to schools nationwide, Madison ranks below the 30th percentile in math and reading skills. One out of six students qualifies as learning disabled. A typical year sees about 300 incidents of crime and violence (see distribution in Fig. 1). The most common violation of the Student Code of Conduct at Madison is fighting. As one Assistant Principal explained, sixth graders are immature, "they look at each other—they fight." (TCPR & AP, 2000)

Simply outlawing violence in schools doesn't work. In reaction to nationwide outrage at highly publicized gun incidents, many school districts instituted a Zero Tolerance policy wherein any weapon infraction could result in a compulsory lengthy suspension or expulsion. Madison's principal Thelma Davis contributed to the controversial report "Opportunities Suspended: The Devastating Consequences of Zero Tolerance and School Discipline" (TCPR & AP, 2000) which rebuts this approach. The report concludes:

> The increasing use of [zero tolerance] practices throughout the country is denying thousands of children opportunities for education, and alienating more from the educational process. Moreover, data clearly shows that minority students are frequently far more harshly disciplined than their white counterparts for similar, or less serious, offenses. Zero Tolerance is unfair, is contrary to the developmental needs of children, denies children educational opportunities, and often results in the criminalization of children.

Victim Services of Miami were originally invited into the school by the school social worker in order to provide bereavement groups because many children at the school lost caregivers to AIDS and homicide. Many of the children we served were from these bereavement groups. Others were from the severely emotionally disturbed group and many more were referred by the school social worker who had identified that they had overwhelming trauma in their lives

Types of Crime and Violence
at Madison Middle School

☐ Property damage

■ Alcohol/Drugs

▨ Weapons

☐ Disorderly conduct

☐ 5%   ■ 3% ▨ 2%

■ Personal violence

■ 8%

▨ Fighting and
Harrassment

▨ 77%

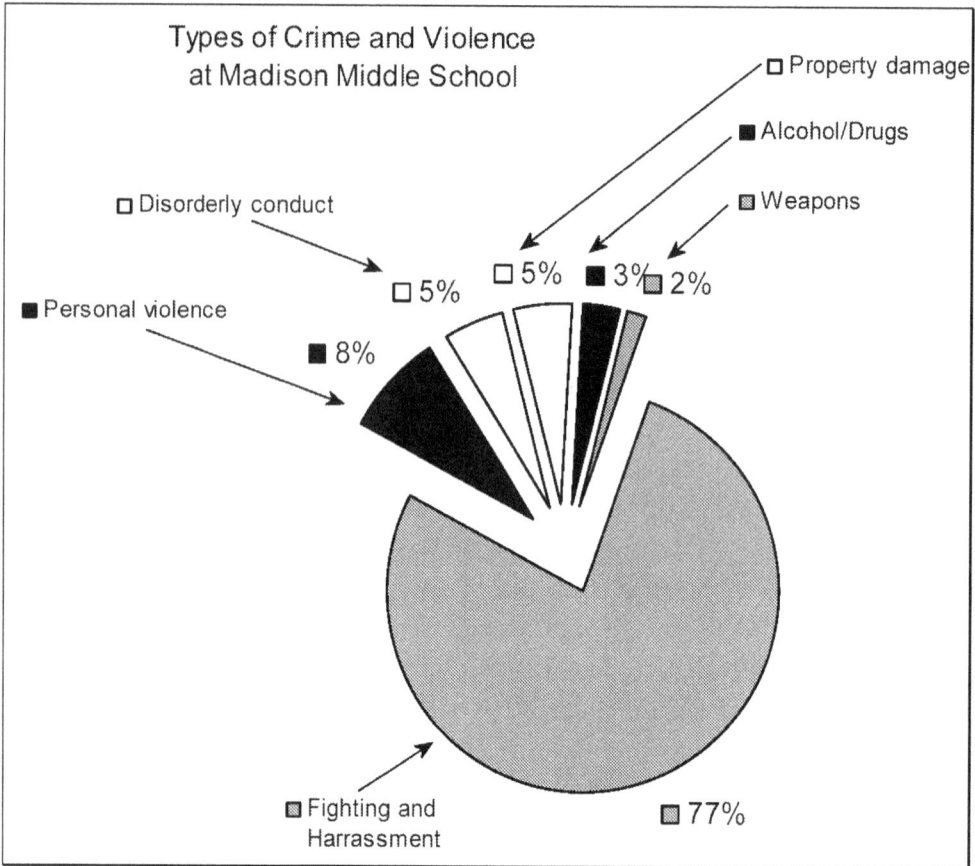

Distribution of Crime and Violence at Madison (Fig. 1)
Source: www.schools-data.com

## Trauma and Childhood

Our understanding of trauma in children is strongly informed by the work of Ricky Greenwald, Ph.D. of Mt. Sinai Medical Center. In his book *Trauma and Juvenile Delinquency: Theory, Research, and Interventions* he documents the role of trauma in conduct disorder, antisocial behavior, and delinquency. This book also highlights the success of trauma-informed and competent services for at-risk youth.

Another influence in our thinking is Bruce Perry, M.D.'s research on child maltreatment. Perry explains how persisting fear can alter the developing child's brain. Specifically, these early traumatic events contribute to schizophrenia in patients who have a genetic predisposition. The neurodevelopmental costs of adverse childhood events can no longer be ignored. In *The Cost of Child Maltreatment: Who Pays? We All Do* (Franey, Geffner & Falconer, 2001) Perry states that children with PTSD as a primary diagnosis are often labeled with Attention Deficit Disorder with Hyperactivity (ADD/HD), major depression, oppositional defiant disorder, conduct disorder, separation anxiety or specific phobia. Underlying this is the idea that the brain forms in a use-dependent fashion. Childhood is a critical and sensitive period for brain development; disruptions at these times may lead to abnormalities or deficits in neurodevelopment. Experiences of over-activation of important neural systems during sensitive periods of development can manifest in several ways, including:

- Malorganization and compromised functioning in:
    - —humor, empathy, attachment and affect regulation
    - —being insensitive to any replacement experiences later in life, including therapy
- Being stuck in hyperarousal or dissociation:
    - —males tend to manifest hyperarousal
    - —females tend to manifest dissociation
- Fear becomes a trait:
    - —Very easily moved from mildly anxious to feeling threatened to being terrorized
    - —Maladaptive emotional behavioral and cognitive problems arise

## Treatment Approach

Traumatic Incident Reduction was the primary approach that we utilized. The only difference in how it was delivered to children was that we incorporated some sort of craft activity that the children would engage in as they recounted their traumatic incidents. Beadwork turned out to be the most popular activity for both girls and boys. It seems that pairing a relaxing, right brain activity, with an initially distressing right brain activity, lowered the arousal for the children through recounting rapes, beatings and homicides.

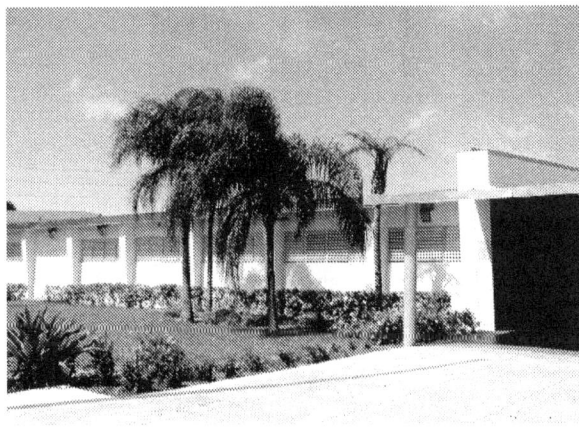

*Madison Middle School*

Since we changed our measurements for the third year of the grant, the following data only represents the 2003 academic year. Two factors limited our impact on the student body to thirty-five students during year three. Funding was the primary limiting factor and secondarily that children had to have three out of four of the aforementioned domain risk factors. It should be noted that the Madison Middle School program is strictly a pilot project—whose purpose is to see what outcomes are possible—rather than a research driven project.

## Measurement Scales Utilized

Our treatment approach used four different scales to pre- and post-test the children on the impacts that trauma was having on their lives.

- Child Report of Post-traumatic Symptoms (CROPS) (Greenwald and Rubin, 1999) – with a clinical cut-off of 19
- The Depression Self-Rating Scale (Birleson, 1981) – 13
- Self-Concept Scale for Children (Lipsitt, 1958)
- Youth Coping Index (McCubbin, Thompson, and Elver) – acceptable range -91.8 to 95.4

## Case Summaries

Two of the thirty-five cases are highlighted here in brief:

Case #1: A 12 year-old Hispanic female—victim and witness of abuse, in the Florida Department of Children and Families system who underwent 14 hours of individual treatment with TIR and 12 hours of group therapy over a seven month period:

| Measurement | Pre-test | Post-test |
|---|---|---|
| Student Form | 19 | 0 |
| Depression SRS | 15 | 0 |
| Self-Concept Scale | 88 | 109 |
| Youth Coping Index | 53 | 102 |

After treatment, she wrote:

> "The changes I've had ever since I started sessions here is I don't think I have to be perfect any more to impress my friends. Ever since I stopped trying to be perfect, my friends said I have become a better artist and a better friend. And I have become a better person as well."

Case #2: A 15 year-old African-American female—victim of sexual abuse, drug abuser and runaway. Underwent 15 hours of individual treatment with TIR, labeled as Oppositional Defiant

| Measurement | Pre-test | Post-test |
|---|---|---|
| Student Form | 39 | 6 |
| Depression SRS | 18 | 2 |
| Self-Concept Scale | 47 | 102 |
| Youth Coping Index | 71 | 128 |

After treatment, she wrote:

"I know that my behavior changed. My attitude, my ways and also my language. And the service help me a lot because I don't do bad things anymore or don't follow people. And my grades in school has improve a lot with As, Bs, Cs in conduct."

## Results

First, I need to emphasize again that this was not a research project; the statistics gathered were in the interest of practicing responsibly. Children measured in the study all had symptoms of traumatic stress. Although there was no attempt to diagnose for PTSD, many of the children were above the PTSD cutoff on the Student Form and Depression Self-Rated Scale. Both scales show children significantly below the PTSD cutoff levels following treatment, as the following charts indicate:

Average Results from Pre- and Post-Tests (N=35)

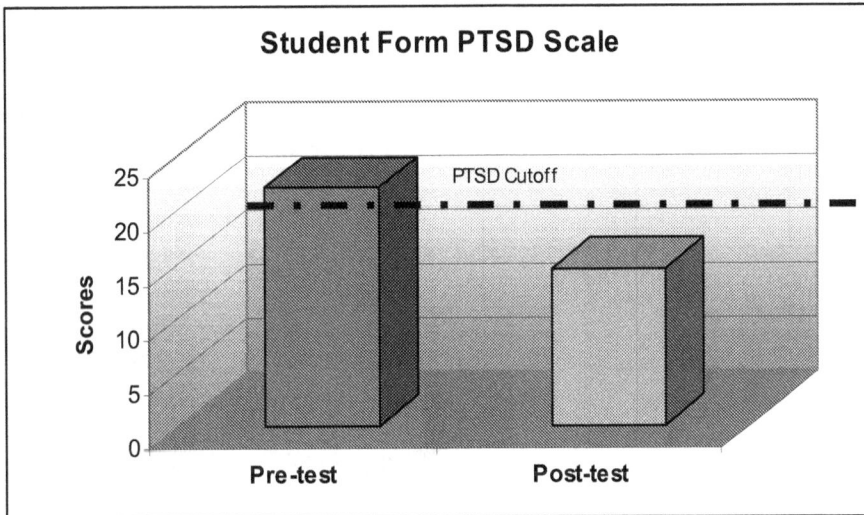

## Depression Self-Rating Scale

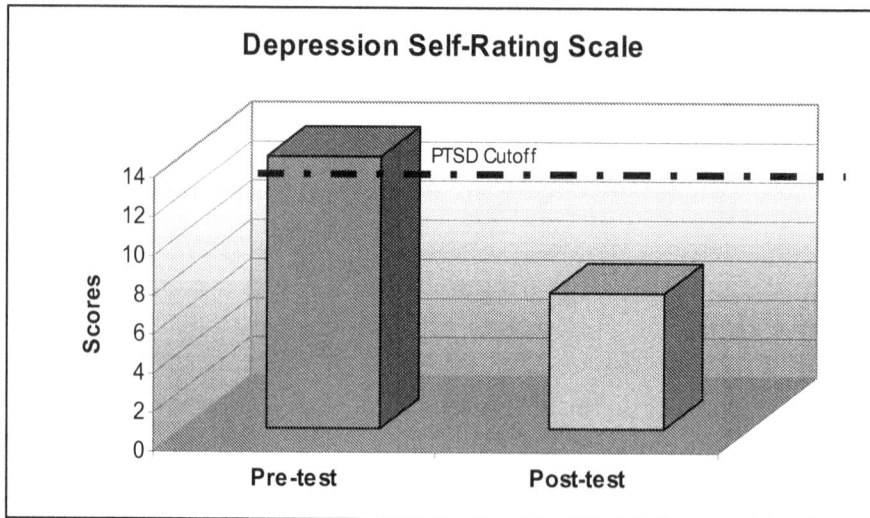

## Self-Concept Scale

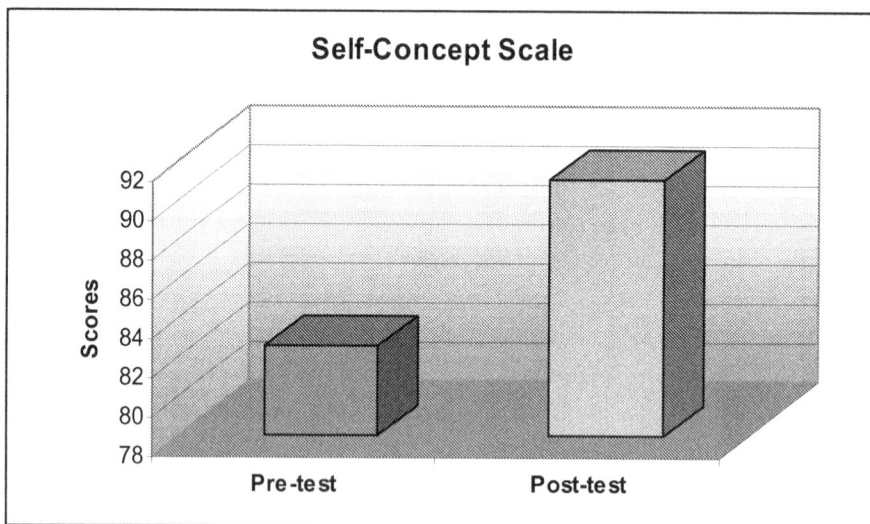

[Ed. Note: average data for YCI was not available at time of press.]

## Summary

We have heard from the school social worker at Madison Middle School that our trauma focused program is the most effective service received by her students. She has reported to me that the children who went through our program are doing better academically and with behavior at school and at home. I see that this program will offer a deeper solution to stopping the cycle of violence and helping youth move out of the category of "At Risk" and into truly resilient people.

## References

Depression self rating scale [DSRD] (1981). Birleson P. IN: Corcoran K & Fischer J (2000). Measures for clinical practice: A sourcebook. 3rd Ed. (2vols.) NY, Free Pr. V.1,Pg.535-536

Self concept scale for children [SC] (1958). Lipsitt LP. IN: Corcoran K & Fischer J (2000). Measures for clinical practice: A sourcebook. 3rd Ed. (2vols.) NY, Free Pr. V.1,Pg.617-618

Youth coping index [YCI] (1995). McCubbin HI; Thompson A; Elver K. IN: Corcoran K & Fischer J (2000). Measures for clinical practice: A sourcebook. 3rd Ed. (2vols.) NY, Free Pr. V.1,Pg.628-631

Franey, K., Geffner, R., and Falconer, R., Ed. (2001). The Cost of Child Maltreatment: Who Pays? We All Do. Family Violence and Sexual Assault Institute, San Diego, CA.. http://www.fvsai.org

Greenwald, R. & Rubin, A. (1999). "Brief assessment of children's post-traumatic symptoms: Development and preliminary validation of parent and child scales". *Research on Social Work Practice, 9,* 61-75.

Greenwald, R. (2002) Trauma and Juvenile Delinquency: Theory, Research, and Interventions. Haworth Maltreatment and Trauma Press.

Civil Rights Project, The & Advancement Project (2000). "Opportunities Suspended: The Devastating Consequences of Zero Tolerance and School Discipline Policies." Delivered at National Summit on Zero Tolerance (2000). The Civil Rights Project, Harvard University. http://www.civilrightsproject.harvard.edu/research/discipline/opport_suspended.php

**Victim Services – The Trauma Resolution Center** (TRC) in Miami, Florida is a unique and pioneering trauma services delivery model for trauma survivors who often are plagued with mental health and substance abuse problems following experiences of crime and violence, but are typically denied services in the mental health, substance abuse, and victim assistance worlds because their needs do not "fit" with how those providers have been trained. The TRC serves all types of people who have experienced traumatic events – such as rape, domestic violence, witnessing violence and/or murder, torture, kidnapping and numerous other types of human to human violence – in an integrated and empowering short-term series of group and individual sessions that specifically address trauma and the range of its mental health, substance abuse, and victimization related personal impacts. A trauma services model termed "Traumatic Incident Resolution" (TIR) is used by TRC and applied to each staff member who completes the TIR process him or herself prior to beginning to counsel clients using the TIR model to accomplish trauma resolution. A host of the client's additional personal and life style issues related to the traumatic event(s) are also addressed by TRC staff through advocacy and case management. With a full time staff of 16 that treats approximately 800 clients per year, in addition to providing basic advocacy/case management services for over 800 more clients per year, the TRC is an extremely economical human services program model with tremendous bang for the buck. It is a very transformative approach to trauma services design and delivery that merits national attention and application in a wide variety of communities.

Susan Salasin, Public Health Advisor
Prevention and Program Development Branch
Center for Mental Health Services, Substance Abuse and Mental Health Services Administration (SAMHSA)

# 6 Active Ingredient Study: Preliminary Findings

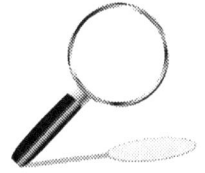

## by Joyce Carbonell, Ph.D.

[Ed. Note: The following transcript is excerpted from the plenary session of Joyce Carbonell, Ph.D. at the 9th Annual Conference on Metapsychology in 1995.]

In 1994, TIR, V/KD, EMDR, and TFT were investigated through a systematic clinical demonstration (SCD) methodology at Florida State University. This methodology guides the examination but does not test the effectiveness of clinical approaches. Each approach was demonstrated by nationally recognized practitioners following a similar protocol, though their methods of treatment varied. A total of 39 research participants were treated, and results showed that all four approaches had some immediate impact on clients and appear to also have some lasting impact. The paper also discusses the theoretical, clinical, and methodological implications of the study.

## Introduction

I'll start this presentation with some background about the project, and I'll tell you why I got involved. I run the University Crisis Management Unit and I work with the Critical Incident Stress Debriefing Team. I also work with some of my fellow mental health workers in town and together we formed the Community Crisis Response Team. I've worked with Vietnam vets, people on death row, and rape victims. I've never had a traditional sort of clients in any sense of the word. My clientele were almost always in some sort of trauma, crisis, or involved in a very ongoing trauma. That is, they were sentenced to death, they had a warrant signed, they were on trial, they were in an abusive relationship, or they were raped and their rapist was at large. I also work with people who have more traditional traumas such as Vietnam veterans and law enforcement officers.

For years, Charles Figley and I have both been very interested in stress and trauma in very different ways. Charles is particularly interested in compassion fatigue, Vietnam veterans and some traumatized groups. Since we both taught at the same university, we eventually got together. As a result of leading the trauma study group, we developed this project. When you look through the literature and you get some idea of how frequent and how common trauma is, it's really appalling. The lifetime prevalence rates of PTSD are incredibly high; more for some groups than others (Christensen & Jacobsen, 1994). For example, 25% of those exposed to any stressor and 35% to 92% of those who were raped have traumatic stress. Clearly not everyone gets traumatic stress.

Some people can go through numerous experiences and not develop symptoms and yet others will develop them.

## Prevalence Rates

Prevalence rates became part of our curiosity also. Could we not only find a way to treat it, but could we find a model for finding out how traumatic stress gets induced? Why do some people seem to be more likely to have it happen while some people don't seem to have it happen? It happens in traumatic bereavement, in people molested as children, and in 65% of those who experience some kind of non-sexual assault. We tend to forget people like your average mugging or burglary victim.

For example, my in-laws' house was recently burglarized. They had lived out in the country for years in a rural area. They loved it and felt incredibly safe. They finally sold their small business so they could go on vacations. After their first vacation, they came home and found it ransacked. They did not leave the house empty since then. Someone is always there now, and it has made a terrible dent in their lives. And you may say "It was just things that got stolen," but what really got stolen from them was what happens to a lot of traumatized people: any sense of safety, trust, and belief in other people. There are tons of traumatized people out there who will probably never be officially diagnosed as having PTSD and never seek help for the simple reasons that they don't want to, they don't know how, they don't know the process, and they don't want to be labeled. Vietnam veterans can obviously fit into this category. A much forgotten group is prisoners-of-war from World War II and veterans of that war. Some veterans interviewed recently about the battle of Iwo Jima (50 years ago from that time) were clearly suffering badly at the slightest mention of what they had seen or done. Studying the data confirmed the importance of searching for the model of how traumatic stress gets induced.

## Incidence Rates

Charles and I were just so amazed at the amount and tenacity of trauma that people suffered, that we decided this was something that we would continue to pursue. For example, burn patients have a very high rate of trauma as nurses and physicians know. The article from the aforementioned cited statistics points out that "We have done a very good job in recent years of documenting that people suffer." We document it quite well. Yet what happens is that we tend to do very little about it. There are all kinds of literature documenting who suffers and how they suffer.

The *Journal of the American Medical Association* published a review of 150 studies on PTSD and the highest success rate was 20% with an average of 30 hours of treatment. Even then, they weren't claiming to completely eliminate the symptoms of PTSD. Of course the other impetus behind this was that we realized that most treatments are slow and somewhat ineffective. "ED-75" is the Effective Dosage for which 75% of the people get relief. There are charts for drugs and all kinds of treatments with an ED-75 level. This is rather frightening both in terms of time and cost.

In Kopta's study (1994), they reviewed charts where clients had filled out questionnaires for having the presence of symptoms after therapy sessions. Then they charted out how many therapy sessions it took per symptom to resolve. Assuming a basis of $75/hour, they charted how it cost per symptom. "Crying easily," the cheapest for example, required an average of 22 fifty-minute sessions before clients felt relief. On the other hand, "Worrying too much" costs approximately $9000. There is some older research that indicates that your degree doesn't particularly make you a more effective therapist. Paraprofessionals do just as well in therapy, and yet certainly doctoral-level psychologists charge a lot more.

> *There is some older research that indicates that your degree doesn't particularly make you a more effective therapist.*

## Brief Treatments

Contrary to the frightening costs mentioned above, we found lots of clinical claims of being able to treat PTSD in short periods of time. These came from people like Milton Erickson, Neurolinguistic Programming people with Visual Kinesthetic Disassociation (V/KD), and then TIR practitioners. The other approach which came to the forefront recently [in the early 1990s] was EMDR. According to some sources, EMDR has become the most widely researched among current treatments. Another treatment which is probably the least known and least well accepted method is Thought Field Therapy (formerly known as the Callahan Technique). We ended up with these four approaches to PTSD, some of which were more publicly accepted than others.

All of them were very different from each other except in the one respect that they all seemed to be able to cure. That is they seemed to make people feel better in short periods of time. They were not like the aforementioned study where it took 67 hours to make clients "feel better about the future". Can you imagine if there was truth in advertising when clients came in? You would have to say "You're feeling lonely? That will be 86 sessions". My advice would be to buy a dog; dogs are wonderful for feeling lonely. We convened a panel of experts who advised us on these different treatments. We can thank Teresa Descilo for getting us interested in TIR. She approached Charles, who was talking about compassion fatigue, and assured him that she never had any!

## The Study

We had some concerns. (1) It had to be something that there were at least 500 people trained in. (2) There had to be some clinical evidence of its effectiveness. (3) An international group of trauma experts with which we consulted had to agree that this would in fact be an appropriate treatment.

We devised something we called a systematic clinical demonstration. This is not your traditional methodology. Our goal was not to compare these four treatments and say which one was best. The goal was to find the Active Ingredient: What was making these things work? Why did these things work? We hoped that if we could find that Active Ingredient that we could design a model of how traumas and phobias are induced in people and how they happen. We don't have a particularly good model for that. We have some, but we still can't explain why some people do and some people don't [have traumatic stress].

Phobias are one of the strangest manifestations of traumatic stress. The worst snake-phobic I'd ever seen had no one else in her family who was ever afraid of snakes, had never had a particularly nasty experience with snakes, couldn't remember the last time she had ever seen a snake, and couldn't remember a time when she wasn't afraid of snakes. That's not particularly uncommon with phobias. Phobias are very specific. Have you ever known anyone with a chair- or table-phobia? No. There is a certain subset of things that people develop phobias about.

Many studies fail that try to look at treatments because they take people inexperienced in the treatment, have them do the treatment, and then say, "See, it didn't work." Or they'll compare two treatments with therapists that are well-trained in one but not in the other method. We wanted to see the very best for each of these. We essentially contacted the originators of each of these particular approaches and invited them to come to Tallahassee. The originators from all four of these come from no place other than California (audience laughs).

> *What we wanted to do is see the very best therapists for each of these treatments.*

We invited these people out. TIR was our first group of practitioners, and because they were our first group, it was a little strange. I offer our sincere apologies to Ragnhild Malnati, Teresa Descilo, and Frank A. Gerbode, for the problems. Our equipment broke down; there were problems with our research personnel, and so on. We handled these before the following groups came to work with us. For NLP, we had Ed and Maryanne Reese, who had originally studied with Richard Bandler and they were using V/KD. For EMDR we had Steve Silver and Roger Solomon. Although we invited Francine Shapiro, she could not come because she had committed months before to do a Level 2 workshop. For TFT, it was Roger and Joanne Callahan.

## The Clients

We advertised in the paper that we were looking for clients that had trauma stress. We gave interviews and we had blurbs on public radio. A few clients literally drove up after hearing it. We rarely turned anyone away. The therapists were not given a choice of clients; the clients were randomly assigned. We would schedule as many as we thought we could. Most of our clients had not experienced just one highly stressful event but as many as 30 highly stressful events. 98% of these clients had prior therapy, frequently unsuccessful. Many of them had been dumped by their therapists. We excluded people who were mentally retarded, minors, blatantly psychotic, drug abusers, and those people on psychoactive medications. To be included in our study, they had to have at least one active symptom of PTSD or phobia but not necessarily a formal diagnosis. Ages ranged from 18 to 58 and averaged 40 years of age.

Clients had to agree to be treated during specific dates and times. There was a week for each treatment: TIR was done for a week in September; V/KD was done for a week in October; EMDR was done for a week in November; TFT was done for a week in December. We did not give people a particular treatment that they requested. They were just assigned to the next group to come in; they did not self-select. Our clients came into these treatments knowing nothing about them except that they were brief treatments known to be effective for traumatic stress. We left description of the technique to the therapists to avoid any bias.

These are the types of traumas from clients that we saw: abusive relationships, problems with parents, moves, loss, death, accidents, imprisonment, child abuse, rape, war veterans, divorce, and phobias. Most people had multiple problems. The phobias that we saw were very, very severe. They were phobias that impinged on people's lives.

## Treatments in Action

Clients who were actually seen varied by treatment randomly selected for them. TIR therapists saw everyone who walked in the door, for which we thank them. One V/KD client rejected the therapists because he wanted TIR instead. EMDR rejected 8 of approximately 14 clients. The EMDR therapists decided that many people were not ready for EMDR and that they needed prior preparation of therapy. Also, they were concerned about abreactions to EMDR and only having a week available for treatment. TFT saw 15 out of 15 clients. We did not invite our therapists to reject our clients. We were in fact dismayed when our therapists rejected our clients. It was not what we had in mind, but they did.

Sometimes the number of clients was partly related to the average length of treatment. The TIR people had quoted two hours as the average length of treatment, though they had to allow more variance. We eventually let the therapists schedule the clients themselves, it seemed so much safer. V/KD takes close to the same amount of time as TIR. It was hard to determine the length of treatment for EMDR, because there were so many rejected clients who were never treated. TFT asked us to schedule no more than 40 minutes per client, so we were able to schedule considerably more clients. 71% of all clients were female. This may be a function of the fact of the gender statistics on mental health problems. Women are much more likely to report depression and anxiety disorders whereas males are much more likely to be diagnosed as personality disorders and substance abuse disorders. The overall rates are the same, but the breakdown in categories are different.

All of these seemed to work; you can't ask me which one did better. For TIR, the average length of a session was 71 minutes. V/KD clients were seen for 49 minutes per session, EMDR in 53 minutes, and TFT in 32 minutes. The largest number of treatments was 4 sessions since there were only 4 days in a week.

They are all so different. One of our issues became, what is the Active Ingredient? They all worked, by the way. All of our clients who were treated felt better on the SUDs [Subjective Units of Distress] scale. Some people say, "Well those subjective ratings don't mean anything."

One of the important issues is: *me* telling you that you should feel better is not particularly relevant if *you* don't feel better. How many have you ever been to physicians or had surgery and you go back in and say "Well, but it's not working, it doesn't feel good." They say "Well, it should." Then they sort of blame it on you; you must be doing something wrong. Then they want you to go away and not come back. I like to hear what clients have to say. All of the clients felt subjectively better after treatment.

> ***All of the clients felt Subjectively better after treatment.***

## Narration and interpretation

Let me tell you a little about what we're trying to theorize about these treatments. V/KD and TIR involve the client narrating the incident. EMDR and TFT truthfully require very little verbalization. EMDR in its most basic level does not require much in the way of verbalization on the part of the client. TFT requires virtually nothing, if they don't want to tell the therapist what it is, they don't even have to. On the other hand, in TIR you do no interpretation for the client. You do not say to your client: "That's probably related to something that happened in your childhood." You would not presume to know what happened; you would not in fact interpret those things for the person. TFT does the same thing; they do absolutely no interpretation. They do not interpret for you why you are afraid or why you have this chronic recurring memory.

V/KD will often interpret for the person: "Maybe what you know now, that that person [in your past] didn't know then, is that it's not your fault." In EMDR, they do what is called cognitive interweaving. They will in the course of it interweave an explanation for the person. One woman got really upset every time an ambulance came by. She was actually distressed because during the cognitive interweaving he said, "It's not your fault that your father died; he had the heart attack." She snapped back "I know that." She did know that and she didn't feel guilty.

# Theories about the treatments

In some ways the interpretive and non-interpretive treatments have a striking resemblance in what they do. One of our theories is to try and figure out why all of these varied and disparate treatments work. One of the theories that we are playing with is that all of these behaviors and fears are maintained, sometimes operantly. In the case of the woman with the snake phobia who couldn't go out the front door it was operantly maintained. In part, by her husband who went out and checked for snakes everyday. It's maintained perhaps in two ways in that she's maintaining his behavior also which is protective. Many of these things are probably classically conditioned. Remember Dr. Gerbode's model of things getting associated one by one [see Chapter 1]. These things seem to be classically conditioned yet to some extent operantly maintained. They are maintained by the environment, although classically conditioned to get there. This may explain why they are hard to break into. Maybe what all these treatments do is break into that loop. I also firmly believe that anxiety also has a physiological component. Very few people feel causatively anxious without having any physical sensation of anxiety, even though they don't always label it. So you have anxiety cognitions and you have physiological symptoms and there are probably some other things. Just looking at those two, they are kind of linked to together. It seems that some of these treatments are breaking into that loop or linkage.

In TIR, they keep exposing themselves to the "conditioned stimulus". What never happens? The stimulus doesn't get reinforced or interrupted. In the beginning, some of the people are starting to get very upset and they cry and they get distressed. But then as they keep going, it extinguishes. In a normal therapy session when a person gets that upset, you interrupt it. So they never get to go and experience that condition stimulus to find out that the conditioned response is never going to happen again. In TIR, that cognition gets to keep going and going. So TIR and V/KD (to some extent) seem to break in at the cognition level. The person gets to keep experiencing that cognition. When you think about it, it makes perfect sense. In traditional therapy, when a client cries what do we do? We try to stop them because we don't like it. They never get to find out that the next thing isn't coming. The reason you see that rise in emotion because they're expecting it. And eventually what happens is that it doesn't come and it extinguishes.

EMDR and TFT seem to do something very different in that they seem to be interrupting at the physiological level. One of the things that they seem to accomplish is that the clients lose their physiological sense of anxiety.

None of these treatments destroy the memories. But the clients seem to then have it as a memory as opposed to an ongoing experience. What EMDR and TFT tend to do is interrupt it at a physiological level so the person can have a cognition but not have that funny feeling. These treatments seem to break in at very different points.

We keep referring to these things as traumatic memories for people. But I actually think that all of these things we are treating are ongoing experiences. Lots of us have memories; I had six car accidents in two years, and I can remember all of them. On the other hand, we saw a client who had only one car accident with minor injuries, and at the very thought of tires squealing or cars getting close she would have basically a full-blown panic attack. For some people, and we don't know why, those things tend to remain as an ongoing traumatic experience. [Ed. Note: see Gerbode's Traumatic Incident Network in Chapter 1 for one possible explanation.] What all of these treatments seem to be able to do is move traumatic incidents into the realm of a memory. They don't look back and say "My goodness isn't that wonderful that I was raped?" But they can look back and say "I was raped. That was sad." But it's not a constant refueling of that [sadness]. These people have these sort of chronic traumatic experiences related to those memories. These treatments seem to break into this at different points. I can't say which treatment is better. Some may be more appropriate for some people more than others.

Our client who said "I never got to talk" would probably like TIR much better. On the other hand, we had clients who didn't want to talk, who were happier with one of the other treatments for a variety of reasons. They were either not willing to tell what it was or didn't want to. But then again, we didn't give clients a choice of treatments. It seems to me that what we are doing with these treatments is taking this conditioned response and separating it from that stimulus. Some of them seem to break in on that cognitive level and some of them break in on the physiological level.

The treatments seemed to work in spite of the tremendous variations between therapists' personalities. Most of our clients had been in pain for a very long time. What they wanted was relief. They cared much less about the therapist than we did. In fact, some of them actually didn't like the therapists and would say so. On the other hand, they admitted that they felt better. Some of them a week later could not remember who their therapist was. If nothing else, it tells you that therapists are fairly unimportant; clients don't care about you.

My traditional notion of therapy has always been that you're watching people get better. You can't force the person to get better. We have a distinct advantage in that most people come to therapy because they do either want to get better, to change something or fix something that's making them uncomfortable. We can give them the tools, we can watch them, but in some ways it's not us, it's them.

For more information about the **Active Ingredient Study** see
http://www.fsu.edu/~trauma/promising.html

## Selected References

Christensen, A. & Jacobson, N. (1994). Who—or what—can do psychotherapy. *Psychological Science*, 5, 156-167.

Kopta, S.M., Howard, K.I., Lowry, J.L., & Beutler, L.E. (1994). Patterns of Symptomatic Recovery in Psychotherapy. *Journal of Consulting and Clinical Psychology*, 62, 1009-1016.

Recordings of this lecture available on the
*Beyond Trauma: Companion Disc.*
(A compilation of MP3 audio files playable on all computers)

**Loving Healing Press**
**www.LovingHealing.com**

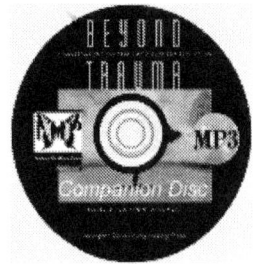

# A Systematic Clinical Demonstration of Promising PTSD Treatment Approaches

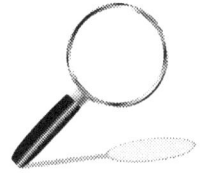

## 7

By Joyce L. Carbonell and Charles Figley

### Florida State University

## Abstract

Traumatic Incident Reduction, Visual-Kinesthetic Disassociation, Eye Movement Desensitization and Reprocessing, and Thought Field Therapy were investigated through a systematic clinical demonstration (SCD) methodology. This methodology guides the examination, but does not test the effectiveness of clinical approaches. Each approach was demonstrated by nationally recognized practitioners following a similar protocol, though their methods of treatment varied. A total of 39 research participants were treated and results showed that all four approaches had some immediate impact on clients and appear to also have some lasting impact. The paper also discusses the theoretical, clinical, and methodological implications of the study.

The authors may be contacted via carbonel@darwin.psy.fsu.edu and cfigley@mailer.fsu.edu respectively. Reprinted with permission from *TRAUMATOLOGY*, 5:1, Article 4, 1999.

## A Systematic Clinical Demonstration of Promising PTSD Treatment Approaches

Efforts to find an efficient and effective treatment for post-traumatic stress disorder (PTSD) have been slow. The field of traumatology has emerged nevertheless to claim the attention of researchers and clinicians trained in the traditional disciplines of psychiatry, psychology, social work, and nursing and practicing in those fields emerging more recently. Family therapy, psychobiology, neuroscience, and pharmacology are examples. The research designs, statistical methods, and highly effective measurement devices from each of these fields have melded into the new field of traumatology. The last and most significant frontier for this new field to identify is a set of treatment approaches that lead to a significant reduction in the presenting problems of a set of clients.

The set of clients of most interest to traumatologists is traumatized people. One or more of a wide variety of traumatic stressors traumatized them. Examples include combat-related stressors, violence-related stressors, stressors associated with loss, and other sources.

This is the second in a series of reports on the "Active Ingredient Project" at Florida State University. An earlier article (Carbonell & Figley, 1996a) described the project in general terms, but the focus was on the therapist traumatized by events outside the office (the murder of a spouse) and an additional on line article (Carbonell & Figley, 1996b). This report will provide a description of the purpose, methodology, the first published results of the study, and a discussion of the results. Later reports will describe individually, and in more detail each of the four approaches examined here.

A recent article Green (1994) notes what many traumatologists now conclude, that we need to move beyond reiterating that traumatic events cause PTSD. Green calls for greater efforts to understand the basic processes to avoid and eliminate PTSD. She suggests that scientists move away from simply documenting the presence of PTSD. Rather, there should be more emphasis on studies of treatment, prevention, and basic etiological processes that will enhance our understanding of how human beings struggle to adapt to severely adverse environments, and how we can help them.

## Managed Care Pressures

In addition, the demands of managed care have forced both practitioners and managers to face an intriguing set of facts. Specifically, although traditional psychotherapy takes time and motivation on the part of both the practitioner and client, managed care, and the economics associated with it, intensifies the need for efficient and effective treatments.

Partly as a way of illustrating the time commitment involved in therapy, Kopta, Howard, Lowry, & Beutler (1994) conducted archival research on the files of 854 patients who had more than 62 symptoms of acute distress, chronic distress, or characterological disorders. The team reviewed the records of a year or less of once-weekly psychotherapy sessions. Each client completed a symptom questionnaire at various points in his or her treatment program to indicate his or her recovery progress. The team calculated the "effective dose (ED) of psychotherapy" for 50 per cent of psychotherapy cases. The ED was defined as the point at which the patient is more similar to normal functional persons than to dysfunctional peers. Thus, an ED50 is a kind of break even point in psychotherapy treatment. The investigators also calculated the ED75 or the effective dosage of 75 per cent of cases.

Kopta, et al. (1994) reported that for the most common acute-distress or chronic-distress symptoms. One hundred twenty sessions (120 hours) of treatment were required to relieve 75 percent of the depressed clients from the symptom of "worry too much." Given the average hourly cost of psychotherapy at full billing of $75 per 50-minute session, the estimated cost would be a staggering $1650 to reach the effective dosage (or number of psychotherapy sessions) for 75% of clients with depression.

Further, Kopta et al. reported that clients seeking significant clinical improvement with the symptom of "crying easily" require 22 sessions (50-60 minutes per session). Thus, it would cost would be $1600. In contrast, for 75% of clients with anxiety seeking a similar level of relief for the symptom of "feeling tense" require 106 sessions at a cost of $7950. Thus, the time and cost required today, utilizing standard methods of psychotherapy practice, to effective treat (secure clinical improvement in) a wide variety of psychological problems is enormous. There appears to be no hope in sight for reducing these numbers.

## Current State of Clinical Traumatology

It is not surprising that the treatment of PTSD, which encompasses many of the symptoms reviewed by Kopta, et al. (1994), takes so long. A recent review of current treatments of PTSD, Solomon, Gerrity, & Muff (1992) conclude that the effectiveness with which we treat PTSD is less than sterling. Their meta-analysis of all published studies found that pharmacotherapy as well as psychotherapy through behavior, cognitive, psychodynamic and hypnotherapies were effective. However, no treatment approach reported even a partial success rate greater than 20% after 30 hours of treatment. Based on the Kopta, et al. (1994) study, there should be greater efficacy beyond 30 hours of treatment. Indeed, it would seem plausible that most clinicians would expect PTSD clients to be more difficult to treat than the presenting problems reviewed by Kopta, et al. (1994), a notion supported by Seligman (1994) who noted that only "marginal" relief is possible for those diagnosed with post-traumatic stress disorder.

Traumatized clients appear to require a special amount of emotional energy, both from the therapists and from themselves, to overcome the barriers imposed by their own fear and lack of hope (Figley, 1997). Clients often work hard to recall nearly all the details of the traumatic event and its aftermath. For many clients, these recall sessions may cause as much or more suffering than the original traumatic experiences when considering the anxiety experienced prior to and during the therapy session. Those who have also experienced a tangible loss are especially vulnerable (Figley, Bride, & Mazza, 1997). And, as noted earlier, the effort often does not eliminate the symptoms caused by the traumatic experiences. It is not surprising so many who suffer from PTSD have abandoned hope of finding relief from their PTSD symptoms, and feel no hope of finding a permanent cure.

There have, however, been claims from the clinical community that apparently brief and effective treatments are available. Though theses treatments not yet proven scientifically, perhaps clinicians responsible for treating clients presenting with PTSD are in a good position to provide sound hypotheses regarding treatment approaches that work and those that do not. Not only does their clinical work demand the most effective approach, but also their continuing education activities expose them to a variety of techniques. Although unorthodox in approach, perhaps these untested treatments deserve further examination.

Among the challenges of evaluating these new treatment approaches are questions such as: How do we know this is not just the latest in a series of fads that come and go, leaving disappointed clinicians and frustrated clients? How does one know if dramatic initial gains last over time?

One of the more challenging criticisms of brief treatment approaches or any other that can be replicated empirically is that they can be taught to, and used by paraprofessionals. Some argue that nearly anyone who is trained in these treatment methods can become effective—irrespective of formal education and credentials. Indeed, there are a large number of persons without formal mental health training and education who have attended training sessions in many of these approaches. There is genuine concern that the quality of care is significantly decreased when performed by non-professionals (Nietzel & Fisher, 1981).

But, several meta-analytic studies of comparing the effectiveness of psychotherapy between professionals and paraprofessionals seem to indicate that the quality of care is not diminished by the use of paraprofessionals. Durlak (1979), for example reviewed 42 studies and found most could not confirm that treatment provided by professionals is superior to that provided by paraprofessionals. Although Durlak found one study showed professionals to be superior the reverse was found in 12 other studies. Regarding measurable outcomes, Durlak concluded, "professionals may not possess demonstrably superior clinical skills when compared with paraprofessionals. Moreover, professional mental health education, training and experience do not appear to be necessary prerequisites for an effective helping person" (p. 80).

Later meta-analysis studies confirm this conclusion (Berman & Norton, 1985; Weisz, Weiss, Alicke, & Klotz, 1987). These studies are further supported by meta-analyses that have demonstrated a lack of overall effects of professional training and experience. Across 475 studies of psychotherapy outcome, Smith, Glass & Miller (1980) found no relationship between years of therapist experience and therapy outcome. Shapiro and Shapiro (1982) who reviewed 143 studies later confirmed this. Although part of the differences can be explained (Christensen & Jacobson, 1994), Shapiro & Shapiro acknowledge that it is more important for the field of psychotherapy to be overly modest than overly confident in their claims. And, it seems that concerns over quality of care provided by paraprofessionals may be unfounded.

## The Research Program

Recognizing the mental health problem of traumatic stress and the lack of adequate methods of preventing and treating PTSD, a program was developed to examine and evaluate innovative methods of treating traumatic stress. Six goals were described: (1) identify the most promising psychological treatments of traumatic stress; (2) investigate these treatments utilizing a systematic clinical demonstration (SCD) methodology (Carbonell & Figley, 1996b) which expands on suggestions from Liberman and Phipps (1987) ; (3) collaborate (via the internet) with a large group of local, national, and international clinicians and scholars interested in the goals of the project to help investigate the treatments; (4) identify the active ingredients in each treatment and that appears to be successful in climinating traumatic stress symptoms; (5) develop a testable, theoretical model that accounts for the process by which people become traumatized, display traumatic stress reactions, and recover from the traumatic experiences and no longer display these reactions; and (6) develop and test clinical guidelines for treating unwanted traumatic stress reactions.

## Significance

This study represents a first step in evaluating innovative treatments that are used by some practicing clinicians and paraprofessionals, but are as yet unexamined under controlled conditions. It represents an attempt to bring together both the academic and clinical communities in evaluating such approaches. In contrast to conventional psychotherapy research, the SCD methodology is not meant to compare the various treatments, and thus does not necessarily meet the criteria proposed for empirically validated treatments (Chambless, et al., 1996), although it does meet some of those criteria. But, it is hoped that such initial research will stimulate interest and encourage others who might ignore these unusual and relatively untested approaches to begin additional research on treatments that seem promising, however unorthodox they appear.

# Method

## Selection of treatment approaches to be evaluated

The first goal of the project was to select treatment approaches for evaluation. To select the approaches the researchers sought the advice of a large number of practitioners and researchers worldwide. The project and its goals emerged from discussions among these colleagues through a specially established Internet forum, currently called the Traumatology Forum [2], which now has a membership of approximately 900 individuals from over 16 countries. To select innovative and promising methods of treating symptoms of post-traumatic stress, a survey was sent to 10,000 members of the Internet consortium, InterPsych (Figley, 1994). They were asked to nominate treatments that were extremely efficient, and could be observed under laboratory conditions.

In addition to soliciting through the Internet, the authors contacted hundreds of clinicians to solicit treatment nominations. An advisory board made up of traumatologists who are part of the Traumatology Forum examined nominated treatments, regardless of how the nomination was obtained. From these discussions four approaches were identified for the initial phase of investigation: Traumatic Incident Reduction (TIR), Visual Kinesthetic/Disassociation (V/KD), Eye Movement Desensitization and Reprocessing (EMDR), and Thought Field Therapy (TFT). Each of these treatments was in use clinically, but had at that time a paucity of research examining their

---

[2] Current address is "traumatic-stress@freud.apa.org" To join, send a message to owner-traumatic stress@freud.apa.org

effectiveness. Other approaches were noted, such as various exposure-based, behavioral and cognitive treatments.

## Investigation

The second goal of the project was to investigate treatments using a systematic clinical demonstration (SCD) methodology (Liberman and Phipps, 1987). Since the treatments had not been examined extensively, we established an initial trial design that simply measured observed changes in the client. In medicine, phase I trials are primarily concerned with safety, not efficacy, and focus on determining deleterious side effects, optimal treatment doses, and so on. This phase may require as few as 20 patients, but usually no more than 80 Phase II trials are small-scale studies of treatment efficacy and safety and designed to closely monitor each patient for adverse events. Phase III trials are conducted after efficacy is reasonably established and involves hundreds of patients (Pocock, 1983). Our adaptation of the clinical trial methodology chiefly involves modification of the Phase I and II research components. In addition to the time and money saved, phase III trials can then focus on only the most promising treatment approaches for PTSD (Carbonell & Figley, 1996).

The innovators of each of these approaches were invited to form a treatment team to participate in the research project. To participate, the innovators were required to send a treatment team to our laboratory for 7 to 8 days. These teams treated clients provided to them during that period of time and under the conditions imposed by the research design. Each of the four innovators of the treatment approaches provided a team of clinicians to participate. Each treatment approach is described below briefly.

Trauma Incident Reduction (TIR). The TIR treatment team was the first scheduled to participate (mid September). Gerbode (1988) described TIR as a Rogerian-based treatment method that follows a carefully crafted protocol. He asserted the result is a rapid method of traumatic memory retrieval that is both humane and empowering. The client, with little coaching from the therapist, can recall critical information about the nature and consequences of the traumatic events.

Visual Kinesthetic Disassociation (V/KD). This approach was represented by the second treatment team to participate in the study (mid October). V/KD, which is a component of Neurolinguistic Programming (NLP), is practiced internationally to eliminate phobia and trauma symptoms. It employs, among other methods, a "fast phobia trauma cure procedure," developed originally by Richard Bandler, which asks the client to focus on the causal origin of the traumatic stress. It establishes a 3-place dissociation method that reportedly enables the client to eliminate all affect associated with the stressor (MacLean, 1986; Einspruch & Forman, 1988; Andreas & Andreas, 1992).

Eye Movement Desensitization and Reprocessing (EMDR). This approach was represented by the third treatment team to participate in the study (mid November). Clinicians report EMDR is a "miracle treatment" for its rapid treatment of a variety of phobias and PTSD symptoms.

Similar to the V/KD treatment approach, clients are asked to focus on a goal for treatment that not only eliminates the unwanted symptoms, but also generalizes to other areas (e.g., self-confidence). Clients then are asked to address certain circumstances associated with the traumatic event (e.g., associated thoughts and feelings) while they focus their attention on a rhythmic stimulus. Most often this stimulus is the therapist's fingers waved at a certain rate to produced lateral eye movement (Shapiro, 1989; Shapiro, 1995).

Thought Field Therapy (TFT). This approach was represented by the final treatment team to participate in the study (mid December). TFT, formerly was known as the "Callahan Technique," reportedly involves rapid elimination of a wide variety of unwanted symptoms. It combines both cognitive reprocessing and use of circulatory fields (meridians) within the body. The treatment appears to have roots in applied kinesiology (Blaich, 1988). The client is asked to concentrate on the stimulus that causes the symptom (thought field) while performing a prescribed "algorithm" of actions. The innovator claims the procedure directs various "thought fields" in a way that eliminates the symptoms ("perturbations") permanently. Unlike the aforementioned approaches, TFT can be used over the telephone, through audio and videotapes or to treat groups of people simultaneously (Callahan, 1991; Callahan & Callahan, 1997).

## Pre and Post Study Symposium

As part of the philosophy that this research should be a community-wide, multi-disciplinary, and multi-professional effort including both practitioners and clinicians, two symposia were held for each of the treatment approaches. (Halpert, 1966) noted that many research findings that could improve clinical practice are either unknown because they are never published or never read by clinicians; thus the symposiums were one way to expand the body of consumer that would be aware of these innovations and the research.)

Over 130 local area clinicians and researchers attended at least one of the symposia. The first of two symposia for each visiting clinical team was to provide a quick overview of the clinical approach. The researchers provided an overview of the project, which was followed by a presentation by the visiting clinicians. The format included:

    (1) a history of the approach (how and why it was invented);

    (2) a theoretical model of how and why it works;

    (3) a step-by-step procedure for [it]

        (a) how to identify the traumatic stress symptoms,

        (b) how to assess the client's interest and commitment to a successful treatment outcome, and

        (c) a specification of treatment methodology;

    (4) how to identify indicators and counter indicators for treatment;

    (5) how to identify indicators of treatment success;

# Eliminating Posttraumatic Stress Disorder: The Active Ingredient Symposium Series

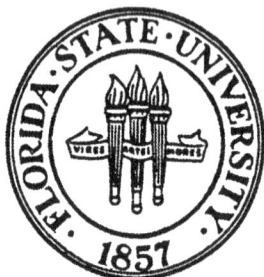

## Coordinated by:
Florida State University
Psychosocial Stress Research Program

## Sponsored by:
Florida State University
Family Institute's Marriage and Family
Therapy Center

Tallahassee Memorial Regional Medical
Center's Psychiatric Treatment Center

Capital Chapter, Florida Psychological
Association

Tallahassee Chapter, Marriage and Family
Therapy Association

National Association of Social Workers
Florida Chapter

Although the PTSD diagnosis is only 14 years old, the syndrome has been identified by other terms since 1900 BC. Despite this long history, no one treatment model or theory is recognized by mental health professionals as the most effective method for diagnosis or treatment. The Symposium Series will spotlight four of the most promising treatment approaches for Post Traumatic Stress Disorder.

Clinicians practicing each of the featured approaches report extraordinary success in a few sessions, compared to traditional methods requiring far longer. The most qualified and nationally known clinicians are invited here to describe their approach and demonstrate its effectiveness of their extraordinary approach under laboratory conditions. The goal of the investigation and the Symposium Series is to identify the most critical factors, the *active ingredients*, in these four PTSD treatment approaches in order to collaborate on a "cure" for all trauma-based disorders.

## SYMPOSIA FORMAT
This series was designed to allow participants an excellent overview of each of the four approaches. Four visiting clinical teams, each expert in one of the treatment methods, will visit Tallahassee during the next months to participate in the Series. Each clinical team will provide an introductory symposium, participate in treatment sessions, and offer a review symposium.

### Introductory Symposia

During the initial symposium, the guest clinicians will present an introduction to their approach, a description of their methods, and a demonstration of the PTSD treatment method.

### Case Treatments

Each clinical team will spend the week following the introductory symposium working with local clients under laboratory conditions. Clients will be carefully screened and tested before, during, and long after treatment. Each client will suffer from at least one traumatic stress symptom that has a negative impact in their daily lives. Psychosocial and Psychophy Biological measures will be taken for all clients, including video and GSR monitoring of the their treatment session and post-session interview. FSU faculty and students will observe the treatment sessions and monitor all clients for six months following treatment.

### Review Symposia

During the review symposium, the guest clinical team will present their cases and discuss their treatment. Resident FSU faculty observers will present their views and critiques. The audience will be invited to join in the discussion. Discussion among these two groups of clinicians as well as clinicians in the audience should ensure a lively and informative 3-hour session.

### Location:

Each of the symposia will be held on Friday afternoons from 2 - 5 p.m. at the Tallahassee Memorial Psychiatric Center, 1616 Physicians Drive, which is located two blocks east of Tallahassee Regional Medical Center.

### Continuing Education Information:

6.0 Hours for Licensed Clinical Social Workers, Mental Health Counselors and Marriage and Family Therapists (Provider Number: CM-245-95)

6.0 Hours for Nurses (Provider Number: 27H0018)

6.0 Hours for Psychologists (CEUs are pending and have been applied for through the Florida Psychological Association.)

The Florida Psychological Association is approved by the American Psychological Association to provide continuing education for psychologists. The APA approved sponsor maintains responsibility for the program.

# SYMPOSIUM SERIES

### The Traumatic Incident Reduction (TIR) Approach

TIR is a Rogerian-based treatment method that follows a carefully crafted protocol that rapidly enables the client in a humane and empowering manner to retrieve important information about the nature and consequences of traumatic events. Presenter: Dr. Frank Gerbode.
*TIR Introductory Symposium, 2 - 5 p.m. Friday, Sept.9, 1994*
*TIR Review Symposium, 2 - 5 p.m. Friday, Sept. 16, 1994*

### Neurolinguistic Programming (NLP) Approach

NLP employs a "fast phobia trauma cure procedure," developed by Richard Bandler, that has the client, similar to the EMDR procedure, focus on the causal origin of the traumatic stress, establishes a 3-place dissociation method that enables the client to eliminate all affect associated with the stressor.
Presenters: Edward and Maryann Reese.
*NLP Introductory Symposium, 2 - 5 p.m., Friday, October 14, 1994*
*NLP Review Symposium, 2 - 5 p.m., Friday October 21, 1994*

### The Eye Movement Desensitization and Reprocessing (EMDR)

EMDR has received wide acclaim as a "miracle treatment" by clinicians internationally for its rapid treatment of a wide variety of phobia and PTSD symptoms. Clients are asked to focus on a goal from the treatment that not only eliminates

the unwanted symptoms, but generalizes to other areas (e.g., self confidence). Clients then are asked to address certain circumstances associated with the traumatic event (e.g., associated thoughts and feelings) while the therapist induces rapid lateral eye movement.
Presenters: Dr. Steven Silver and Dr. Roger Solomon.
*EMDR Introductory Symposium, 2 - 5 p.m., Friday, Nov. 11, 1994*
*EMDR Review Symposium, 2 - 5 p.m., Friday, Nov. 18, 1994*

### The Thought Field Therapy (TFT) Approach

Similar to the previous two approaches, TFT involves rapid treatment of client's various unwanted symptoms through a procedure that asks clients to concentrate on the symptom while performing a carefully prescribed muscle relaxation and stimulation procedure that directs various "thought fields" in a way that eliminates the symptoms.
Presenter: Dr. Roger Callahan.
*TFT Introductory Symposium, 2 - 5 p.m., Friday, Dec. 9, 1994*
*TFT Review Symposium, 2 - 5 p.m., Friday, Dec. 16,1994*

### For additional program information, call 904/644-1588.

Brochure from the 1994 Symposium Series

(6) profiles of treated clients (e.g., presenting problems, demographic profile, time since traumatic event/symptomatic period); and

(7) requirements for training in the use of the approach (e.g., prerequisite education/experience, workshop training requirements).

The purpose of Symposium II was to report the initial results of the study. The clinicians reported the initial results and did presentations of the cases they had seen during the week. The research team presented a panel discussion followed by a question and answer period.

## Procedures

Research Client Recruitment and Screening. Potential clients were recruited through media announcements, and word of mouth "announcements" among local therapists. Potential participants were asked to call a designated number for more information. When they called and identified themselves, the receptionist collected basic information such as their phone number their availability during the treatment period. A member of the research team then returned the potential participants calls to assess their appropriateness for the study. The following criteria were used to initially screen clients.

1.  Participants had experienced life disruption as a result of a traumatic stress symptom and were willing to be videotaped and complete all other aspects of the research for 6 months.
2.  If currently in therapy, participants obtained consent from her/his therapist to participate in the project.
3.  Participants agreed to take no drugs other than those prescribed for mild depression or unrelated to mental health treatment.

If potential participants met the criteria, they were told of the availability of treatment and the times available for treatment. Because each treatment was scheduled for only one week, participants were required to be available during that week. Participants were asked to sign informed consent that a) identified the conditions under which they would be treated (e.g., video taped) and all other requirements (e.g., protocol of the study); and b) agree to be treated during the treatment times and dates at the Clinic. Participants were not required to meet the DSM IV criteria for PTSD, but were required to articulate a trauma or phobia that was interfering with their daily functioning. Participants who chose not to join the study or did not qualify were referred for treatment outside of the study. The participants who agreed to participate and signed the informed consents were scheduled for a pre-testing and assigned to the next available treatment. Participants were assigned to the treatments as they became available. All participants were treated in accordance with APA ethical principles and prior approval for the project had been obtained from the University's Institutional Review Board.

Pre-testing: Each participant received the paper and pencil measures focusing on life stressors and stress reactions, demographic and psychosocial profile, and social support and other resources for managing. In addition, physiological recording was attempted but because of various equipment problems, few data were obtained. The measures to be discussed here are described briefly:

Demographic Information Form (used by the Psychosocial Stress Clinical Laboratory for all clients) - this form provided basic information on each participant.

The Traumagram Questionnaire (Figley, 1989) - this form was a description of each client's individual "trauma history" and was reviewed by therapists before meeting with the clients

The Brief Symptom Inventory (Derogatis & Spencer, 1982) - All participants received the Brief Symptom Inventory (BSI) before and six months after treatment. The BSI is a 53 item self-report inventory in which clients rated their distress of a five-point scale. Subjects are instructed to indicate how much a given problems has bothered them in the past seven days. It is described as a "measure of point in time, psychological symptoms status." The BSI is highly sensitive to change and thus is useful as a tool for pre/post evaluation (Derogatis & Spencer, 1982). The BSI produces nine symptom dimensions and three global indices. The three global indices Global Severity Index (GSI), Positive Symptom Total (PST), and Positive Symptom Distress Index (PSDI) were used in this study. These measures have higher test-retest reliability than any of the individual symptom dimensions available. Research has supported the validity of the BSI as a measure of psychological distress.

Impact of Events Scale (Horowitz, Wilner, & Alvarez, 1979) - The Impact of Events Scale is composed of two separate subscales, intrusion and avoidance. Participants rate each item on a scale of 0 (not at all) to 5 (often) depending on how well the item describes the subject. The items contained in each subscale are summed to form a composite score for each subscale. There is no total score, which combines the subscales. The IES is noted to be useful as a screen for the presence of post-traumatic stress disorder, but does not include symptoms of hyper arousal (Briere, 1997).

Subjective Unit of Disturbance (SUD) rating (Wolpe, 1958): Participants were asked to provide a rating, on a ten-point scale, of their subjective unit of distress (SUD) in regard to their presenting problem before treatment began and immediately after treatment. The participants were also asked to keep a diary on a daily basis for the next six months. A notebook was provided for this purpose and the description of the ratings and instructions were on the inside cover of each notebook. A phone number and name of a member of the research team was also included so that the clients would call with any questions. In addition, a research team member called each research participant on a weekly basis to obtain a SUD rating for the week, to answer any questions and to encourage them to keep their diary.

An attempt was made to videotape each session. The therapist determined session length and the number of visits within the treatment week. Six months following termination, clients were requested to return for follow up testing and were re-administered the instruments described above.

# Results

A total of 51 research participants were pre-tested and assigned to one of the four therapies. Of these 51 subjects 39 received treatment. There were a variety of reasons that the remaining clients did not received therapy in this study. Some declined participation in the study after screening, some were inappropriate for treatment, some did not meet the criteria for the study, and some presented with problems such as uncomplicated bereavement which were inappropriate for the study.

The majority of the participants/clients were female, in both the treated and untreated groups. Twenty-nine females (29 or 77.4%) and ten males (10 or 32.6%) received treatment. Eight females (66.7%) and 4 males (43.3%) did not receive treatment. Thus, 39 individuals were seen in treatment and 12 were not. Clients who received treatment tended to have a higher level of education (16 years) as compared to those not seen (13 years). Those seen in treatment had an average age of 40.8 years, while those not seen had a mean age of 39.1 years. Presenting problems were varied and included traumas such as childhood abuse, combat exposure, criminal victimization, motor vehicle accidents and accidental shooting (See Table 1).

## Length of Treatment

The therapist determined the duration of each treatment session, but the design limited therapy to one week. Therapeutic sessions ranged from four hours (TIR) to 20 minutes (TFT). The average duration of treatment per client, in minutes, was 254 for TIR, 113 for V/KD, 172 for EMDR and 63 for TFT.

Several therapists noted that they saw their clients an additional session event after they thought treatment was complete because they knew that the clients would not have the opportunity to see them again after the week was over.

## SUD Ratings

Although the intent was to ask each subject for a SUD rating, data many of these data were missing. Some of the treatments do not, as part of their procedure, require a SUD rating and thus these ratings were at times forgotten. The lack of a SUD rating does not reflect on the treatment itself, but is a reflection of problems in data collection. In addition, in spite of weekly phone calls/messages, many people did not keep their diaries. For those who did, the ratings demonstrated what could best be described as "slippage" and began to reflect events other than those relevant to the study. For example, a SUD rating would be provided with the description that it has been a "bad day" secondary to things such as car problems, a problem at work, or dismay over the weather. In many cases, there were ratings with no written description, leaving the researchers unable to determine whether or not the SUD ratings in the diary referred to the presenting problem. Given these problems, the SUD ratings reflect pre-treatment ratings and ratings immediately post-treatment.

As noted in Table 2, the SUD scores ranged from a mean of 4.75-6.5 before treatment and from 2.0-5.25 after treatment. It is not appropriate to compare treatment approaches for all the reasons noted earlier. Nonetheless, it appears that EMDR and TFT produced the largest drop in scores.

Results indicate that there was great variability both pre- and post- test SUD scores. The V/KD group had low pre-treatment scores, leaving little room for change. The V/KD therapists treated 9 of the 11 subjects originally assigned to them, as one subject refused treatment upon arrival and the other subject suffered from uncomplicated bereavement and was inappropriate for study. The EMDR group, which treated 6 of 15 subjects also had a low pre-treatment SUD rating. Several subjects in the EMDR group (6) were deemed inappropriate for treatment by the EMDR therapists and most were noted to need more treatment before EMDR would be appropriate. TIR therapists treated all subject who were assigned to them, as did TFT therapists, although one subject did not show up for TFT after having been pre-tested.

## Brief Symptom Inventory

Pre- and post data (Table 3) are presented for subjects who attended the six month follow up. The results are presented for each therapy individually. Scores are presented for each of the three major indices of the BSI, the General Symptom Inventory, the Positive Symptom Total and the Positive Symptom Distress Index. The BSI was scored using psychiatric outpatient norms and pre-test scores were generally at the mean for psychiatric outpatients. It is important to note, for those unfamiliar with the BSI, that the positive symptom total represents the number of symptoms that the client has endorsed, without reference to the level of severity of the symptom. Thus, a pre and posttest score may be the same on this scale, although the severity of the symptoms has changed. The positive symptom distress index, however, reflects both the symptom and the level of distress, and thus would reflect change in symptom severity.

Although changes were relatively small in some cases, there was overall improvement in most cases. As with other measures, there was a great deal of variability among the subjects.

## Impact of Events Scale

Scores are reported (Table 4) for both intrusion and avoidance scales. There are three cutoff points for the IES. A low score is below 8.5, a medium score is between 8.5 and 19 and a high score is over 19. Once again, there was overall improvement in most cases, although not all changes were great enough to move the scores to a lower cutoff. Again, there was a great deal of variability among the subjects.

# Discussion

The purpose of the present study was to explore and examine four brief treatments purported to be efficient, effective treatments for PTSD. Unfortunately, because of problems with client screening and data collection, the study fell short of reaching it goals. Moreover, the nature of the study precludes comparison of the approaches, and such a comparison was never planned. The variety of presenting problems and the varying levels of severity of those problems within each treatment group precluded us from drawing conclusions about the utility of any treatment for any particular type of trauma. Nevertheless, all four of these treatments deserve further study in more controlled conditions and some of these approaches have already been the object of such research.

Although not a comparison of the outcome for each treatment, it is important to determine and examine the similarities between these approaches. If there are similarities, then perhaps there is an "active ingredient" that accounts for the reported success of each of these therapies.

The apparent differences for each of these treatments obscure what may be an important similarity, the client-directed nature of the treatment. Although the treatments vary greatly in their outward appearance, they all require that the client provide and /or direct two important aspects of the treatment. First, in each of the treatments, the control and direct the extent of exposure to the traumatic event they will receive. Second, while creating their own level of exposure to the trauma, each of the treatments provides some intervention, ranging from a form of what could be called unconditional positive regard (TIR) to tapping (TFT). We suggest that the impact of the treatments is to create in the client a relaxation effect at the same time that the client is self-exposing to the trauma. In TIR for example, the method could be described as asking the client repeatedly to expose themselves to their traumatic memories at their own pace accompanied by unconditional positive regard from the therapist. V/KD shares similarities with TIR in that it in-volves multiple "viewing" of the trauma at the client's direction with the support of a therapist. In EMDR, the client also self-exposes while being directed in eye-movements. While the eye-movements are purported to be of importance in a neurological sense, proponents of EMDR also indicate that finger tapping is equally successful, indicating that any success achieved through the use of EMDR is not due to the neurological impact of eye movement, but to some other process. TFT involves the client mentally exposing themselves to their traumatic memories with direction from the therapist on which "meridians" to tap or stimulate. Essentially, in all of the approaches, the trauma is recalled in the presence of relaxation (or if not relaxation, the absence of stress) and thus is not "re-lived" as it is remembered because the negative affect associated with the trauma is not re-experienced with the memory of the event.

Another important similarity is that the client chooses the level of exposure to the stressful materials. Although in both TIR and V/KD, this exposure may be verbalized repeatedly to the therapist, and in EMDR and TFT the exposure is verbalized to a lesser extent, the client still chooses the level of exposure. In addition, all four-treatment approaches seem to lower negative arousal during this self-dosed exposure.

All four of the approaches are highly focused on outcome objectives, exposure based, and client directed both in terms of the selection of traumatic material to be considered and the amount of exposure to the material that they experience. This leads to the hypothesis that the active ingredient may be the simultaneous exposure to the traumatic memory and the reduction in distress. Thus, the client is able to remember the trauma without the negative arousal that previously accompanied the memory of the trauma (Lick & Bootzin, 1975).

Our investigation of these four promising methods of traumatic stress reduction and elimination are far from complete. Yet, these treatment approaches appear to be promising in helping clients remove the most painful aspects of their traumatic memories. It is clear that these treatment approaches are worthy of further study in clinical and laboratory settings to further determine their utility and the active ingredients that account for their apparent effectiveness.

Five aspects of this study distinguish it from others for good or ill. First, an expert panel nominated the promising treatment approaches selected for examination. Second, the developers of each of these treatments were invited to participate in the study and either provided treatment themselves or chose the practitioners. Third, over 100 community practitioners monitored the project through a series of symposia held just prior to and following treatment and data collection. Fourth, the study screened, pre-tested and post-tested the research clients and continues to do so. And, last, the clinical significance and utility were studied.

As noted earlier, this is the second of a series of reports and studies in our research program. Many of the goals of our program were addressed in this report. We have identified four promising treatments and plan to continue monitoring our research clients and conduct follow up testing when possible. We also intend to study other promising approaches, particularly those that purport to eliminate childhood anxiety disorders.

We also plan to continue to utilize the SCD methodology and rely on the consultation of our colleagues through the Internet. In another report we will discuss methodologies utilized in medical and epidemiological research and how the SCD methodology adapts these approaches in an effort to increase the number of clinical innovations investigated. It is hoped that these efforts will decrease the time between discovery or development of a treatment and the initial clinical trial testing, and reduce the cost of psychotherapy research.

Finally, we continue to search for the active ingredients that account for the apparent power of these and other treatments in eliminating or alleviating post traumatic stress symptoms. In doing so, we believe that we will eventually develop a testable theoretical model that accounts for the traumatic stress induction and reduction process. Such a model will lead to the development and testing of clinical guidelines for treatment of post traumatic stress reactions.

Table 1

Presenting Problems

| Problem | Untreated Subjects | | | Treated Subjects | |
|---|---|---|---|---|---|
| | N | % | | N | % |
| Childhood Abuse | 5 | 41.7 | | 15 | 38.5 |
| Death/Loss | 3 | 25 | | 9 | 23.1 |
| Combat/Military | 2 | 16.7 | | 4 | 10.34 |
| Domestic Violence | 1 | 8.3 | | 3 | 7.7 |
| Other | 1 | 8.3 | | 3 | 7.7 |
| Job Related | 0 | 0 | | 3 | 7.7 |
| Sexual Assault | 0 | 0 | | 2 | 5.1 |

Table 2

Pre and Post SUD Ratings by Treatment Group

**SUD Ratings**

| Treatment Group | Pre-Treatment | | Post-Treatment | | |
|---|---|---|---|---|---|
| | Mean | Range | Mean | Range | % Change |
| TIR (N=2) | 6.5 | 4-9 | 3.40 | 3-4 | +48% |
| V/KD (N=8) | 4.75 | 0-9 | 5.25 | 1-9 | -10% |
| EMDR (N=6) | 5.0 | 1-8 | 2.00 | 0-5 | +60% |
| TFT (N=12) | 6.3 | 1-9 | 3.00 | 0-6 | +52% |

Table 3 Pre and Post BSI Scores by Group

## Global Severity Index (GSI)

| Treatment Group | Pre-Treatment Mean | Post-Treatment Mean | % Change |
|---|---|---|---|
| TIR (N=5) | 57 | 48 | 15% |
| V/KD (N=6) | 51 | 43 | 15% |
| EMDR (N=4) | 52 | 43 | 17% |
| TFT (N=8 ) | 44 | 39 | 11% |

## Positive Symptom Total (PST)

| Treatment Group | Pre-Treatment Mean | Post-Treatment Mean | % Change |
|---|---|---|---|
| TIR (N=5) | 52 | 49 | 6% |
| V/KD (N=6) | 52 | 46 | 11% |
| EMDR (N=4) | 55 | 42 | 23% |
| TFT (N=8 ) | 41 | 39 | 5% |

## Positive Symptom Distress Index (PSDI)

| Treatment Group | Pre-Treatment Mean | Post-Treatment Mean | % Change |
|---|---|---|---|
| TIR (N=5) | 57 | 48 | 16% |
| V/KD (N=6) | 49 | 40 | 18% |
| EMDR (N=4) | 54 | 42 | 22% |
| TFT (N=8 ) | 51 | 41 | 19% |

Table 4 Pre and Post Impact of Events (IES) Scores by Group

**Intrusion Scale**

| Treatment Group | Pre-Treatment Mean | Post-Treatment Mean | % Change |
|---|---|---|---|
| TIR (N=5) | 24.0 | 19.0 | 21% |
| V/KD (N=6) | 22.0 | 11.5 | 47% |
| EMDR (N=4) | 24.3 | 12.0 | 50% |
| TFT (N=8 ) | 12.6 | 11.3 | 10% |

**Avoidance Scale**

| Treatment Group | Pre-Treatment Mean | Post-Treatment Mean | % Change |
|---|---|---|---|
| TIR (N=5) | 33 | 17.8 | 47% |
| V/KD (N=6) | 16.7 | 12.5 | 25% |
| EMDR (N=4) | 15.8 | 11 | 30% |
| TFT (N=8 ) | 13.8 | 11.6 | 16% |

Traumatology, 5:1, Article 4, 1999

# References

Andreas, S. & Andreas, C. (1992). Neuro-Linguistic Programming. In S. H. Budman, M. F. Hoyt, and S. Friedman (Eds.), The First Session in Brief Therapy, pp. 14-35. New York: Guilford.

Berman, J. S. & Norton, N. L. (1985). Does professional training make a therapist more effective? Psychological Bulletin, 98, 401-407.

Blaich, R. M. (1988). Applied kinesiology and human performance, Collected Papers, International College of Applied kinesiology.

Briere, J. (1997). Psychological Assessment of Adult Posttraumatic States. Washington, D.C.: American Psychological Association.

Carbonell, J.L. & Figley, C. F. (1996a). When trauma hits home: Personal trauma and the family therapist. Journal of Marital and Family Therapy, 22, 53-58.

Carbonell, J.L. & Figley, C. F. (1996b). Systematic clinical demonstration methodology: A collaboration between practitioners and clinical researchers. TRAUMATOLOGYe (on line serial), 2(1). Available www: http://rdz.stjohns.edu/trauma.

Callahan, R. J. (1991). Why Do I Eat When I'm Not Hungry? New York: Doubleday.

Callahan, R. J. & Callahan J. (1997). Thought Field Therapy. In C. R. Figley, B. Bride & N. Mazza (Eds.), Death and Trauma. Washington, D. C.: Taylor & Francis.

Chambless, D.L., Sanderson, W.C., Shoham, V., Bennet Johnson, S., Pope, K.S., Crits-Christoph, P., Baker, M, Johnson, B., Woody, S. R., Sue, S., Beutler, L. , Williams, D.A. & McCurry, S. (1996). An update on empirically validated therapies. The Clinical Psychologist, 49, 5-18.

Christensen, A. & Jacobson, N. (1994). Who--or what--can do psychotherapy. Psychological Science, 5, 156-167.

Derogatis, L. R. & Spencer, P. M. (1982). The Brief symptom Inventory: Administration, scoring and procedures manual-I. Baltimore: Clinical Psychometric Research.

Durlak, J. A. (1979). Comparative effectiveness of paraprofessional and professional helpers. Psychological Bulletin, 86, 80-92.

Einspruch, E. L & Forman, B. D. (1988). Neuro-linguistic programming in the treatment of phobias. Psychotherapy in Private Practice, 6(1), 91-100.

Figley, C. R. (1989). Helping Traumatized Families. San Francisco: Jossey-Bass.

Figley, C. R. (1994). Survey of members of the Interpsych consortium of newsgroups. Internet distribution, January through May, 1994. Archives, Traumatic Stress Forum.

Figley, C. R. (1997). Preface (pp. xxi-xxvi). In C. R. Figley, B. Bride & N. Mazza (Eds.), Death and Trauma. Washington, D. C.: Taylor & Francis.

Figley, B. Bride & N. Mazza (Eds.) (1997). <u>Death and Trauma</u>. Washington, D. C.: Taylor & Francis.

Gerbode, F. (1988) <u>Beyond psychology: An introduction to metapsychology</u>. Palo Alto: IRM Press.

Green, B. L. (1994). Psychosocial research in traumatic stress: An update. <u>Journal of Traumatic Stress</u>, 7 (3), 341-362.

Halpert, H. P. (1966). Communications as a basic tool in promoting utilization of research findings. <u>Community Mental Health Journal, 2</u>, (3), 231-236.

Horowitz, M., Wilner, N., & Alvarez, W. (1979). Impact of Event Scale: A measure of subjective stress. <u>Psychosomatic Medicine</u> 41: 209-218.

Kopta, S.M., Howard, K.I., Lowry, J.L. & Buetler, L. E. (1994) Patterns of symptomatic recovery in psychotherapy. <u>Journal of Consulting and Clinical Psychology</u>, 62, 10009-1016.

Lick, J. & Bootzin, R. (1975). Expectancy factors in the treatment of fear: Methodological and theoretical and theoretical issues. <u>Psychological Bulletin</u>, 82, 917-931.

Liberman, R. P. & Phipps, C. C. (1987). Innovative treatment and rehabilitation techniques for the chronically mentally ill. In W. Menninger & G. Hannah (Eds.), <u>The chronic mental patient</u>. Washington, D. C. : American Psychiatric Press.

MacLean, M. (1986). The neurolinguistic programming model. In F. J. Turner (Ed.). <u>Social Work Treatment: Interlocking theoretical approaches, 3rd Ed.</u>, pp. 341-373.

Nietzel, M.T. & Fisher, S. G. (1981). Effectiveness of professional and paraprofessional helpers: A comment on Durlak. <u>Psychological Bulletin, 89</u>, 555-565.

Pocock, S. J. (1983). <u>Clinical trials: A practical approach</u>. New York: John Wiley & Sons.

Scott, M. J. & Stradling, S. G. (1994). <u>Counseling for Post-Traumatic Stress Disorder</u>. London: Sage.

Seligman, M. E. P. (1995). <u>What you can change and what you can't.</u> New York: Knopf.

Shapiro, D A. & Shapiro, D. (1982). Meta-analysis of comparative therapy outcome studies: A replication and refinement. <u>Psychological Bulletin, 92</u>, 581-604.

Shapiro, F. (1989). Efficacy of the eye movement desensitization procedure in the treatment of traumatic memories. <u>Journal of Traumatic Stress</u>, 2 (2), 199-223.

Shapiro, F. (1995). <u>Eye movement desensitization and reprocessing: Basic principles, protocols and procedures</u>. New York: Guilford.

Smith, M. L., Glass, G.V. & Miller, T. I. (1980). <u>The benefits of psychotherapy</u>. Baltimore: Johns Hopkins University Press.

Solomon, S. D., Gerrity, E. T., & Muff, A. M. (1992). Efficacy of treatments for posttraumatic stress disorder. Journal of the American Medical Association, 268: 5, pp. 633-638.

Weisz, J.R., Weiss, B, Alicke, M. D. & Klotz, M. L. (1987). Effectiveness of psychotherapy with children and adolescents: A meta-analysis for clinicians. Journal of Consulting and Clinical Psychology, 55, 542-549.

Wolpe, J. (1958). Psychotherapy by reciprocal inhibition. Stanford, CA: Stanford University Press.

# 8 Researching PTSD: Going for the Cure

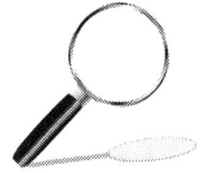

## Mary Sykes Wylie

Voltaire once wrote that history was "little else than a picture of human crimes and misfortunes," but not until our own era of mass communication did it become practically impossible to escape constant bombardment by bad news. Wars, natural disasters, industrial catastrophes, highway carnage, crime, terrorism, sexual abuse, rape, domestic violence all make trauma a horrible and daily leitmotif of the 20th century. The saving grace to this bleak picture, however, is that a culture steeped not only in the ever-present images of trauma but also in the concepts of mental health is becoming more aware that even during the course of ordinarily uncatastrophic lives, things will happen that have the power to shock and wound perfectly sane and well-adjusted people to their very core.

An estimated one-half to three-quarters of the general population in the United States has been exposed to an event that's severe enough to result in diagnosable Post-Traumatic Stress Disorder (PTSD). How many traumatized people actually develop PTSD is another question, but the number is probably high. According to various studies, 47 percent of rape victims suffer from PTSD three months after their assault, for example, while 25 percent of those who lost a relative to an accident or violence are diagnosed with it, along with 31 percent of Vietnam War veterans at some point in their lives and up to half the victims of natural or manmade disasters. In short, as many as 25 percent of the people exposed to the traumatic events that are becoming endemic to modern life can be expected to develop full-blown PTSD as a consequence. These people our neighbors, our friends, our families, ourselves are thus vulnerable not only to the horrifying flashbacks, nightmares, irrational fears, sudden angers and emotional numbness that officially define PTSD, but to the less dramatic anxieties, depressions, substance abuse, phobias and personality disorders that may follow in its trail.

Yet while the epidemiology of PTSD has been exhaustively documented, the remedies are not remotely so obvious. Even as treatment methods for PTSD and claims for their effectiveness proliferate, hard outcome research randomized, controlled studies that meet the gold standard set by mainstream academic psychologists is sparse. In 1992, National Institute of Mental Health researcher Susan Solomon discovered that of 255 English-language articles describing "effective treatments" for PTSD written since 1967, only 11 were randomized, controlled studies the rest were mainly anecdotal. And of the 11, 5 were pharmacological studies showing little or no improvement in PTSD. Of the remaining 6 studies of behavioral and cognitive techniques the most

improvement came when a combination of both modalities was used in a study of 66 rape victims; nearly 70 percent no longer showed symptoms of PTSD after three months. Since then, two
or three other controlled studies of cognitive-behavioral therapy with rape victims have shown
very good results. There are also several controlled studies of PTSD treatment by Eye Movement
Desensitization and Reprocessing (EMDR), a fairly new approach that is so controversial that the
validity of research done on it is still vigorously debated. But with these meager exceptions, a
therapist looking for solid research evidence for treatments routinely used for PTSD won't find
much on which to hang an intervention.

Of course, if therapists had to wait for empirical validation for their favorite model or the ad
hoc mix-and-match methods they customarily use before treating clients, their ranks would
probably shrink to a tiny remnant of cognitive-behaviorists seeing mainly phobics leaving the rest
of the field almost entirely to medication-prescribing psychiatrists, who wouldn't be doing much
actual psychotherapy either. But most therapists don't wait for the latest outcome study, with its
tables, graphs, scales, sub-scales, inventories and t-scores. Faced with a desperate client who isn't
improving, they are more likely to plunge ahead in an old-fashioned spirit of what-the-hell em-
piricism, and try almost anything in any combination, from the old standards of the psychology
texts to the latest workshop sensation.

Academic researchers are appalled by what looks to them like treatment promiscuity and by
clinicians who behave like impressionable groupies, serially infatuated by a long line of performance artists, magicians and mountebanks. Like weary and beleaguered defenders of reason in a
world overrun by superstition, research psychologists argue that psychotherapy can have little
standing as a reputable science of healing until its methods have been empirically demonstrated to
work. These critics of the clinical *vox populi* argue that the alleged "miracle cures" popping up in
the field like dandelions after a spring rain are merely artifacts, piggybacking on the unmiraculous
facts of therapy in general. Researchers point out, for example, that clients tend to improve no
matter what the clinical model; the positive effects of their own hopes and expectations of improvement, the novelty of the new technique, the therapist's undivided attention, empathy,
suggestion and personal talent are often indistinguishable from the specific impact of a particular
method. Without the rigors of a scientific method that controls for all these "confounding" issues, how is it possible to know whether something new and different really is something new
and different, or just the same old stuff tarted up in new duds?

The lack of academy-approved, hard validation for most therapy methods has not stopped
thousands of clinicians from using whatever methods they think will help their clients, with most
generally feeling at the end of the day that they have probably helped somebody, somehow. But
PTSD seems different. Faced with clients who have experienced, or committed, the worst enor-
mities life has to inflict, many therapists lose heart and the confidence that they have much to
offer. Listening to the harrowing stories of their traumatized clients, clinicians themselves can
succumb to the pernicious contagion of PTSD symptoms the intrusive images, nightmares, exaggerated startle reflex, irritability, sense of helplessness and confusion. Furthermore, people whose

lives have been shattered by war, child abuse, political imprisonment and torture their symptoms often compounded by substance abuse, failed relationships, job instability are among the most compelling and demanding clients therapists ever meet. "Working with vets, I am confronted daily by suffering of an intensity that no person should ever have to experience," says Jean Steinberg, a psychologist with the PTSD unit of the Department of Veterans Affairs in Salisbury, North Carolina. "It can take months and months of work before you see an impact on even one chronic nightmare."

Severely traumatized clients challenge not only the effectiveness of standard therapies but their very relevance as if the ordinary stuff of clinical interventions were somehow trivial in the face of suffering beyond the pale of any neat diagnostic category. Kate Sorensen, director of Trauma Relief Services, a private agency in Flagstaff, Arizona, recalls that several years ago, she had nearly burnt out on therapy after working for two years on a Navajo reservation with traumatized children and adolescents. "There were just too many heart-breaking stories," says Sorensen, "and although I sometimes felt helpful, I practically never felt I could do enough for [kids] in such desperate need."

Sorensen remembers one incident in particular a 13-year-old boy referred by the local school for fighting and doing poorly in school, whose father had shot himself in his truck three years before while his son sat next to him in the passenger seat. Sorensen says that she knew this was at the base of his problems, but that "he didn't really want to talk about it, and I didn't want to poke around when I had no confidence in what I was doing. I'd been taught the usual things counseling, reflective listening, some cognitive-behavioral techniques but I really didn't have much sense of how to help somebody who obviously had suffered an enormous wound. What was I going to say to this boy, 'When your dad blew his brains out as he sat next to you, how did that make you feel?'"

Yet despite the official pessimism about recovery from chronic PTSD and the void in the literature where effective treatment outcome studies should be, some lucky therapists approach the work with the confidence and enthusiasm of people who know they are making a difference, because their clients are recovering. During the early '90s, while researching a book on compassion fatigue the harder, meaner form of burnout to which trauma therapists are prone Charles Figley, director of the Florida State University Psychosocial Stress Research Program in Tallahassee, Florida, began to meet many therapists who seemed to be immune to the condition. Talking at meetings around the country about the price that PTSD extracts from therapists as well as clients, he discovered clinicians who not only worked regularly with trauma survivors and managed to avoid burnout in the process, but actually found the experience rejuvenating! "I was finding that some therapists, in spite of the fact that they saw a large number of traumatized clients, experienced compassion exhilaration because they were curing people through extraordinary treatment methods." True, the voices of these cockeyed optimists were not coming from official channels not from de jure representatives from Ph.D. psychology programs, academic research institutions, large mental-health facilities (though individual therapists in them might be heard) nor from strict practitioners of only standard methods.

Instead, glowing reports that often amounted to the professional equivalent of born-again experiences were coming from a kind of therapy underground as distinct from the orthodox centers of psychology as the secret, pagan folk religions of the Middle Ages were from the established Roman Catholic hierarchy. In the course of his professional sojourns, Figley would talk to colleagues who reported hearing about methods that had amazing results. Word-of-mouth reports came from people who said they had seen something in a tape or at a workshop, had tried it and their clients had made wonderful progress; now, five years later, they were still using the technique and new PTSD clients were also making wonderful progress.

Indeed, describing their results, these everyday pioneers even dared openly to use the taboo "C" word cure a brazen and immodest claim in the genteel professional establishment. Further, they were doing their cures in record time; instead of the 20 to 300 or more hours of therapy Figley cites as typical for PTSD, it would take them 2, or 3 or 4 hours. And instead of a painful, long, drawn-out process of reliving the trauma, which therapist and client found harrowing (flooding, for example, a therapeutic form of intense exposure to the traumatic material, can elicit severe depression, suicidal thoughts, alcoholic relapse and panic disorders), what Figley was hearing about seemed much less agonizing for both helper and helped.

By tills time, around late 1992, Figley had grown deeply tired of the professional jeremiads about PTSD how prevalent, how damaging, how incurable. There were, and still are, no studies, says Figley, showing that any standard method leads to complete remission of symptoms. "We have failed miserably to treat PTSD," he says. "In most instances, people with chronic PTSD are just giving up, learning to organize their lives around their disability. And the blame for this has to be laid at the feet of those of us who call ourselves experts. We've done a crappy job."

It is a hard assessment, but nobody is in a better position, or less afraid, to make it than Figley, who helped invent the field of traumatology. A Vietnam veteran himself, Figley became aware of a complex and disabling malaise in some of his wartime peers in 1971, when he spent three nights preceding a peace demonstration in Washington, D.C., with a crowd of Vietnam Vets Against the War. A few years later, Figley, then a professor at Purdue, met Shad Meshad, also a Vietnam vet, who was "working the streets," doing impromptu therapy and rap sessions with stressed-out vets. The two fought and won a campaign for federal legislation mandating psychological treatment for Vietnam veterans. In 1978, the book Figley edited, *Stress Disorders Among Vietnam Veterans*, was the first to name and describe the condition he had seen seven years earlier, which would evolve into the formal diagnosis of Post-Traumatic Stress Disorder, included, for the first time, in the 1980 *Diagnostic and Statistical Manual of Mental Disorders* of the American Psychiatric Association.

Figley's career seems dedicated as much to publicizing PTSD as researching it, and he seems to have a genius for getting people's attention, if not endearing himself to the authorities. Not that he cared then or does now. "I've reached a point where I don't give a damn what other people think," he says. Besides writing articles and editing numerous books on psychosocial stress, Figley founded the International Society of Traumatic Stress Studies; the Journal of Traumatic Stress, the first online computer traumatic studies journal; and the Green Cross a fledgling international, Internet-connected organization that mobilizes and dispatches therapists to disaster areas around the world. "Working with Charles is like riding on a roller coaster you never know where he's going next," says Gail Davies, director of the Psychosocial Stress Clinic at Florida State. "About the time you think you've gotten what he's talking about, he's onto something else. His mind just never stops, although it's sometimes hard to understand where it's going."

Typically impatient, Figley decided the normal snail's pace of academic research on PTSD was not acceptable: "What we had been doing wasn't working, and I thought we had to take a different tack, move beyond the university research setting and into the community."

To say Figley was open to the stories he was hearing from the psychotherapy trenches about therapists not only helping, but curing PTSD clients, understates the case. "I wanted to find out what they did, how they did it, how they knew that what they were doing worked. I wanted to catch them being successful, maybe develop out of their communal experience a new theory, a new paradigm. I didn't care what they did or who invented it, I just wanted to know what it was. I wanted to figure out how we could stop the suffering."

Figley also felt that psychotherapy research is past due for an overhaul. "The entire method by which we sanction clinical procedures is flawed beyond repair," he says, because as it now stands, academic researchers don't sanction very much of any practical interest to psychotherapists. So about three years ago, Figley undertook to bridge the gap between research and practice by setting in motion an unusual research project, for which he had only a few modest goals: finding a "cure for PTSD," putting an end to compassion fatigue, stimulating new studies and transforming the entire methodology of psychotherapy research.

In early 1993, Figley and psychology professor Joyce Carbonell, a colleague at Florida State, began to send a "clarion call" to the clinicians of the world for "nominations" of PTSD treatments that practicing therapists found worked the best, regardless of whether they were orthodox, validated, standardized, APA-approved or off-the-wall. To be included in Figley and Carbonell's "active ingredients" project, a systematic clinical demonstration defined as a "user-friendly research methodology that is a collaboration between practitioners and researchers," the methods had to meet several criteria: the approaches had to have been demonstrated to be "extremely efficient," producing within a few sessions an "extraordinary impact on clients' progress in recovering from PTSD," and their effectiveness had to be verified by 200 to 300 licensed or certified clinicians who had actually used them to treat PTSD. Further, the inventors of the methods had to be willing to come to Florida State for a week and publicly show their stuff with assigned clients in a laboratory setting (two to four sessions per client, while being videotaped and watched by area therapists), then stick around for discussions and conferences devoted to uncovering the meaning of it all. Was there an identifiable "active ingredient" common to different successful treatments that made them effective? Would finding this ingredient help develop a theory that explained both the induction and reduction of trauma?

Gathering the nominations was an informal, democratic, if not very systematic, process. The message went out to about 10,000 people via Interpsych, the Internet special-interest traumatology screened the methods for treatment possibilities, plausibility, interest and adherence to the inclusion criteria. Only four methods made the final cut for the scheduled clinical demonstrations. However obscure to the official world of psychotherapy, they had nonetheless all been around in one form or another for at least 10 years one for about 20. Undoubtedly less surprising is that all originate in California. The best known, and probably for that reason the most hotly debated, Eye Movement Desensitization and Reprocessing (EMDR), was developed by psychologist Francine Shapiro. It involves visual, auditory or kinesthetic stimulation while the client focuses on the traumatic material and integrates it. Another chosen method was the relatively conservative Trauma Incident Reduction (TIR), a desensitization and cognitive imagery approach refined in the mid-'80s by Frank Gerbode, a California psychiatrist. In this approach, the client is directed to review a traumatic incident, first silently then aloud, over and over again in the presence of an interested but neutral "facilitator," until arriving at an internal resolution. The third method, Visual Kinesthetic/Dissociation (V/KD), demonstrated by Florida therapists Maryanne and Edward Reese, is related to Neuro-Linguistic Programming (NLP) an approach to human learning and change based on close analysis of verbal, behavioral and sensory patterns developed in the early 1970s by Richard Handler and John Grinder. With V/KD, clients are led through a process of purposeful dissociation, in which they visualize watching a movie or TV program of themselves undergoing the traumatic event. During the process, they imagine communicating with and reassuring their younger, traumatized selves and integrate the entire experience into their present lives. Thought Field Therapy (TFT), possibly the least therapy-like therapy ever invented, created by California psychologist Roger Callahan during the early '80s, requires only that the client think briefly about the traumatic event while specific acupuncture meridian points (supposedly stimulating the body's bioenergy system) are tapped or rubbed. (For detailed descriptions of each approach, see pages 25-29.)

It cannot have been an easy decision for the innovators of these so-called "alphabet therapies" to participate in the project. On the one hand, they had nothing to lose and everything to gain from the study; with the exception of EMDR, none had sufficient name recognition to have much of a reputation, bad or good, and had nowhere to go but up. Even EMDR, with more visibility, but facing more organized opposition, stood to benefit enormously from being included in a high-profile project initiated by one of the world's leading traumatologists in an established university setting. On the other hand, the innovators were aware that their therapies were on trial before an international audience and expected to produce results in one to four sessions for treating unknown, unselected, formally undiagnosed and largely unprepared clients. "It was scary," says psychiatrist Frank Gerbode, whose team demonstrated Traumatic Incident Reduction in the project. "Up to that point, TIR was still relatively unknown, and its reputation rested on how good a showing we had this was it, the showdown at the OK Corral."

In the popular mind, innovators are expected, even required, to have a hard time convincing the world that they have a better mousetrap, even if they really do embattled genius struggling against philistinism is inherent to the myth of creativity. And yet, until recently, psychotherapy has in fact been remarkably open to new ideas. But this traditional attitude of laissez faire is going the way of private practice, as the old freedoms of clinical work sink rapidly under the pressures of the media (which often depicts therapists doing nothing but extracting false memories from helpless clients) and the movement toward stricter practice guidelines, promoted by the burgeoning managed care industry. The current climate of distrust of therapy has made it much harder for innovation to flourish, and much, much harder for innovators to get a hearing.

Roger Callahan, for example, has already undergone his own ordeal by fire, even before heading for Tallahassee. Having had a successful career as a psychology professor, publishing papers and chairing meetings, he suddenly found himself a pariah when he tried to introduce Thought Field Therapy to a wider audience his papers rejected without comment or advice, his requests to give workshops denied, his own practice investigated by the California state board for ethics violations (he had used the word cure in discussing his work) inquiries usually reserved for egregious sexual and financial wrongdoing. ("As a matter of fact," says the irrepressible Callahan, "they closed the investigation, when I did the technique on the investigator and cured her of a phobia.") Last August, at the annual meeting of the American Psychological Association in a workshop Figley led on the "active ingredients" project, after the four innovators had presented their methods, a man in the audience stood up, roundly castigated all four approaches, then pointed a finger at Callahan and said, "As for you, Dr. Callahan, if I were a patient of yours and you were doing that kind of crap to me, I'd sue!" Callahan says he expects militant: skepticism, but doesn't understand why he has faced such relentless hostility and antagonism.

But hostility and antagonism are what innovators can expect to dine on these days, if they become successful and appear to be making a serious dent in the Zeitgeist. Quietly advising moon worship as a psychological treatment might not rouse much interest, as long as it remains buried in the mossy overgrowths of some New Age grotto, but once the word gets out, warning antennae begin to quiver around every psych department in the country. In the battle for legitimacy that an expansive and vastly popular EMDR movement is waging, academics routinely accuse EMDR's Francine Shapiro and her associates of almost every egregious ethical and professional sin in the APA manual, except sexual abuse of clients. EMDR proponents, they say, make unsubstantiated claims about the benefits of the method for personal gain, exaggerate tentatively positive research findings on its behalf while ignoring or suppressing negative reports, prevent verification of EMDR techniques by independent researchers and aggressively market to the public a treatment that has little or no empirical backing.

For example, in one of numerous academic broadsides, "EMDR as Marginal Science," a review of Shapiro's 1995 book about EMDR published in the March 1996 issue of the *Scientist*

*Practioner*, William O'Donohue and Steven Thorp of the University of Nevada in Reno accuse Shapiro of engaging in "pseudo science" and intellectual dishonesty. "We found the explanation of how EMDR works to be a paradigmatic example of the use of scientific-sounding terms to give the aura of science to what is actually babble." Clinicians have picked up on Shapiro, the authors suggest, because "the field of psychotherapy has been none too particular about the evidential credentials of psychotherapies and assessment devices."

Although Robert W. Montgomery, a professor in the Department of Psychology at Georgia State University in Atlanta, had reported favorably on EMDR in a six-subject study he had done with colleague Teodoro Ayllon the previous year in the *Journal of Behavior Therapy and Experimental Psychiatry*, in his review of her book the following year for the same journal, he accused Shapiro of pervasively misrepresenting and misinterpreting research literature, taking a "self-aggrandizing" tone in the text and making "grandiose" claims about EMDR. In an extensive review article, which appeared in the Journal of Behavior Therapy and Experimental Psychiatry, academic critics Jeffrey Lohr, Ronald Kleinknecht, David Tolin and Richard Barrett summed up the results of more than 60 research studies on EMDR, writing that "the results of controlled experimental research provide little in the way of support for EMDR clinical applications."

To many clinicians, and even a few researchers, this attitude embodies the inherent snobbery of the research community. "They [the academic establishment] are holding EMDR to an unfair standard, and requiring more in the way of proof than is normally required, simply because the method doesn't make sense to them," says Temple University psychology professor Jay Efran. Harvard psychiatrist Roger Pitman, an eminent researcher into the psychobiology of treatments for PTSD, once deeply skeptical about the procedure, now believes "the mounting body of evidence in the literature that suggests something about EMDR is effective. . . . Too many people say they have had good experiences with EMDR to completely poo-poo it." But Pitman is still inclined to dismiss the odd identifying feature of EMDR the alternate stimulation (the eye movements, or presumably any other) as "unproven speculation."

The debate about EMDR seems in part an outgrowth of an old quarrel between "town and gown" a de facto class antagonism in the psychology profession that pits higher-status academics against practitioners. Clinicians widely believe that academics regard them as less talented, more often drawn from the lower ranks of psychology students, whose judgment about new methods is more likely to be swayed by "clinical intuition" (i.e. emotionalism) than rational logic and empirical demonstration. "There is a real disdain for clinical work [among researchers]," says Jean Steinberg, who did her graduate work in the prestigious behavioral psychology program at State University of New York at Stony Brook. "At Stony Brook, those of us who wanted clinical positions were steered toward more academic ones. There was a definite sense that clinicians were second-class students and second-class professionals."

What Figley and Carbonell were trying to do with their active ingredients project accommodate the hard rules of science to the infinitely fluid circumstances of life, without fatally compromising the first or misrepresenting the second sounds eminently reasonable. Yet the line between a tyrannical scientific methodology, on the one hand, and a sloppy disregard for all rules of evidence on the other can seem impossibly narrow. Without some standardized, controlled research on therapy techniques, how can clinicians separate the good from the bad from the in-different among scores of therapeutic "breakthroughs" earned aloft by popular appeal? Yet, when the mushy core of most human experience is ignored, science can degenerate into crude scientism an infatuation with scientific style paradoxically undermining the value of research itself. Econo-mist Paul Krugman, in his book, *Peddling Prosperity*, suggests that the problem with most economists is that "they want a subject that is fundamentally about human beings to have the mathematical certainty of the hard sciences," which is a mistake, he writes, because human beings "do not behave in simple, mechanical ways." How much truer are these remarks about the scien-tific attempt to extract unambiguous truths from the almost legendary ambiguities and complexities of psychotherapy?

People who actually do therapy take the command to be more scientific with a grain of salt; they know that therapy today still depends more on relationship than method. "I think Therapy with a capital T doesn't work," says Jay Efran. "People work therapists work and clients work and they find interesting and useful ways to work together. But when we try to turn therapy into a thing, reify it, then I think we are looking for something unreal."

Indeed, the hunger for certainty can actually compromise the search for truth. One psychol-ogy professor at a well-known university research psychology department says that the controlled validity studies he has seen make him cringe. He reports that inexperienced students, who are as-signed to treat the experimental clients for the lead investigators according to rigid manualized treatment protocols, frequently stop using the method being tested after the first session because it seems to have so little relevance to the client's problems and offends the therapist's sensitivity. "Everybody knows there is a lot more going on in the therapy room between two people than is contained in a treatment formula," says this professor. The students end up doing more or less regular, ad hoc therapy, then "write it up as if the manual did the trick. It's practically fraud."

How can a research project be designed that encompasses both scientific research and clinical care, and produces research that means something to members of both worlds? The task of Fig-ley's clinical demonstration was fundamentally to bring the clinic into the laboratory, to demonstrate real therapies on real clients, but in a sufficiently rigorous and controlled way that some empirically valid conclusions (or at least suggested conclusions worth pursuing) could be drawn from the process.

To make the study actually relevant to real practice, Carbonell and Figley bypassed many of the usual academic safeguards. Not only had the investigators chosen treatments largely unknown and likely to raise suspicions in the research community because of their oddness and general lack of orthodox empirical support, they were not very picky about either the provenance or diagnos-tic profile of the client-participants who would be included in the study. When publicizing the project, Carbonell and Figley cast their net wide for subjects, recruiting them from the entire Tal-lahassee area (not limiting the study mainly to university students or known clients of their own colleagues). They sent out their call for participants by radio announcement, newspaper story and word of mouth.

Nor did they demand anything as specific as an actual diagnosis of PTSD, or even particular symptoms. They called only for people suffering the aftereffects of a trauma, whatever that might mean, or a phobia, on the theory that many phobias are embedded reactions to trauma. These were "real clients, self-selected, of incredible variety" says Carbonell.

Ultimately, 51 people were chosen and screened (none were admitted who were retarded, psychotic or taking heavy-duty neuroleptics), tested (various psychological "pen and paper" questionnaires and physiological measurements) and assigned in the order they had come to the next available teams of innovator-clinicians, who were allotted no more than four sessions during one week each in mid-September, October, November and December 1994.

The majority of the participants were women, median age 40, with just under 16 years of education. Although the most common presenting problem comprised unresolved issues from childhood abuse (about 38 percent), the rest were a hodgepodge Vietnam and Gulf War veterans; crime, rape, domestic violence and accident victims; people suffering bereavement or losses (including job loss, divorce, major family health problems, the unresolved death of a parent during childhood); one person who had returned from prison to find his personal network completely gone; and people with various phobias (including a woman terrified of blood, another of snakes but "only snakes falling out of things," says Carbonell, "a snake-from-the-air phobia!").

The project was as rocky, unpredictable and full of unexpected vicissitudes as any typical therapy experience times 51, with the additional complications of the research requirements. In the end, 39 made it through treatment. One male participant, learning that he would be assigned to V/KD, protested that he wanted the one with the waving fingers; assigned to EMDR, he quit anyway because, he said, he "didn't wish to think about" his trauma. Two or three, who had denied using psychotropic medications during screening, later revealed otherwise one, when asked again during the first session if he was taking medications, replied, "nothing except thorazine."

Some seemed to qualify as "traumatized" only in the broadest sense. One man, for example, complained of marital problems, though he said his wife thought he might have been abused as a child; a woman felt anxious about reentering the workplace after a long absence; another couldn't decide whether or not to get out of a family business. Others seemed poor candidates for brief treatment of any kind a couple of clients who appeared to have dissociative disorders, a woman with a driving phobia who was so physically disabled that she would probably never be able to drive anyway. With such a typical, heterogeneous client population, there must have been times when the investigators wished for the nice, homogenous, if strangely exotic, populations of one-phobia-and-nothing-else clients with whom their lucky colleagues conducted normal research projects. One major measurement of improvement, for example, was the Subjective Unit of Distress (SUD) scale a self-report on a 1-to-10 scale of emotional pain and discomfort, obviously susceptible to the vagaries of mood and happenstance provided by all participants before and every day for six months following the demonstration. But how could the investigators determine the impact of treatment, using this scale, on a woman who measured about a 5 on the SUD scale when she began and a 10 (the highest measure of distress) after her first treatment? Upon questioning, the woman admitted she felt much better about her problem, but sitting in the same room for an hour with "that man" (the therapist) had upset her. She had neglected to tell the screener that she did not like men, period. When measured sometime later after the upset of being exposed to the opposite gender had worn off her SUD level had come down to a 3.

And how could the investigators elicit treatment effects when the measurement devices proved so susceptible to personal idiosyncrasy? The participants had agreed to keep daily diaries, receive weekly phone calls from the team and return for a six-month follow-up visit. After being treated, however, some announced they now felt so much better, they no longer needed treatment, thank you very much, nor did they wish to receive phone calls or return to the clinic 17 refused to come back for the six-month "check-up." When Carbonell pointed out to one participant who wouldn't come back that she would forfeit the fee she had paid for treatment (to be returned after the six-month follow-up), the woman replied, "That's okay; it wasn't much money and I don't need it, anyway." One of the later refuseniks, the snake phobic, was herself a therapist.

The diaries produced their own interesting, not always apposite, data. Intended to reveal how the participants rated their trauma or phobia-related SUD on a daily basis, the entries showed a good deal of what Carbonell calls "drift" reflecting the difficulty people have separating the special suffering that brings them to therapy from the ordinary ups and downs of normal life. A participant who came in reporting a history of child abuse might, for example, record for one day, "Felt no fear, no terror pretty good day," while estimating a very high SUD level of 9. When Carbonell asked about this discrepancy, the response was that on that day, she had a flat tire and was two hours late for work.

Both during and long after the project, the innovators grumbled about its research methodology and each other: the clients were too heterogeneous, their symptoms too severe, not severe enough, unsuited to their treatments; there had not been adequate or accurate description of the real conditions of the project; this or that circumstance of the project (which the others didn't have to undergo) prevented them from doing their very best work; there were signs of favoritism (to somebody else); there was not enough time to prepare clients adequately, or there was too much time, leaving them sitting around twiddling their thumbs.

The EMDR clinicians aroused a certain amount of agitation by presumably "picking and choosing" their clients rejecting those they didn't like. Nothing like it, says Steven Silver, one of the EMDR demonstrators; a woman who had been raped was assigned to EMDR, but refused to be treated by a man, so he referred her to the clinic. Others they declined to treat, said the EMDR demonstrators, because they were clearly unsuitable and it would have been unethical and possibly dangerous to continue. One, for example, was a dissassociative client, for whom Roger Solomon, the second member of the EMDR team, felt the treatment might stir up more intense issues and emotions than she could handle without course, if the methods had proven themselves duds at Florida State. Luckily, they did help, though the improvement, like the study itself, resists easy classification and quantification.

According to symptom inventories administered at the beginning of the study, the client participants were typical of the outpatient mental health population. In addition, their average ratings on the SUD scale before treatment ranged from 5.0 to 6.5 (5.0 for EMDR, 5.4 for V/KD, 6.09 for TFT. 6.5 for TIR) moderately high, but not unbearable, degrees of pain. Immediately after treatment of one to four sessions, these ratings came down to between 2 and 3.5 for three of the four methods (2 for EMDR, 2.8 for TFT and 3.5 for TIR). V/KD's average SUD score of 5 was skewed by the assignment to the unfortunate male therapist of the woman who hated men and reported a SUD of 10 right after treatment, even though her actual trauma-related symptoms improved substantially, and V/KD's overall score later dropped to 3. After six months, all the clients' SUD scores were still lower than before treatment, though they had begun to creep up to between 3 and 5 (3 for EMDR, 3 for V/KD, 3 for TFT and 5 for TIR). The increase probably reflects what might be called successive attacks of "bad-day syndrome" the spiking of daily scores related to life troubles that had nothing to do with the presenting problem.

There were other markers of improvement; the symptom inventory, a separate measure from the SUD scale, which averaged around 50 for all participants, came down on average by 7 to 9 points (9 for EMDR and TIR, 7 for V/KD and 8 for TFT). All the clients seem to have improved, some dramatically. One woman, a survivor of childhood abuse, treated with TIR by Teresa Descilo, was so transformed by her first session that nobody on the research team recognized her when she came back for her second appointment. In the few days between, her clothing style, hair color and mood had changed dramatically, and she had gotten a new job. The woman with snake phobia began gardening again something she had not done in years although the downside to her improvement was her husband's disgruntlement at having lost his role as her protector from snakes. Another woman, who had been terrified of going out or staying alone since an assault, could now be by herself without fear and began to enjoy an active social life.

The project bore little resemblance to a typical clinical trial there were no controls (clients assigned to no treatment, for example), diagnoses were not standardized or even particularly reliable, numbers of participants completing the entire process varied substantially among the methods, self-reports in the diaries were idiosyncratic nor was it intended to be a comparative study of which approach worked best. Rather, the project was a pioneering attempt to demonstrate four new methods of treatment on a typical client population within a laboratory setting under as stringent a set of experimental conditions as possible, given very unstringent circumstances.

Even so, "not one client who participated in the project failed to benefit," says Gail Davies, director of the psychosocial stress clinic at Florida State and responsible for administering the project. Did the project find a "cure for PTSD," its purported goal? Figley himself seems to have initially used cure as a bit of energizing hyperbole to nudge the establishment out of its doldrums. Yet quoting the dictionary, he says, a cure is "a method or course of remedial treatment," as well as a "restoration to health." A cure "eliminates troublesome symptoms of trauma," he adds. "Being cured means that clients have gained control over their problems, though they may not have eliminated them completely." Using this definition, some participants do appear to have been "cured" of their traumatic symptoms, even if the approaches did not immediately end chronic depression and loneliness, imbue people with relationship skills they didn't have before, drain away all shame, guilt, anger and self-dislike.

"People want one or two simple formulas to use with everybody, as if all clients were the same," says Davies, who uses all four new methods in her own work. "But no two people are alike and no two experience PTSD the same way and we aren't going to find one quick fix that works for every client. These new approaches are techniques and tools, but not the whole therapy." Nonetheless, says Davies, the so-called "power therapies" seem to "jump start the process of therapy. They move clients along much more quickly through their trauma to a resolution. You can cover more in a single session than in a month of weekly talking."

What about the "common ingredient" Figley had hoped to discover did the project uncover the psychotherapeutic equivalent to Ariadne's thread? A hypothesis has emerged from the study. According to Figley, what all the methods have in common is that they pair the thought of the traumatic event with the sudden dramatic reduction of physiological anxiety, and something like a new neural connection is made between the memory of the trauma and a calmer, more tranquil physical state. Trauma produces a chronic state of "hyperstress," caused by the massive emission of stress hormones (see "The Biology of Fear" page 38); the four approaches all produce a calming effect on the body "hypostress" while the brain is actually mentally reliving the trauma. Says Figley, "The trick is to get the brain focused on the thought evoking the old emotions and feelings, and at the same time introduce something that reduces the anxiety associated with it to switch the program. The idea is to extinguish hy-perstress with hypostress."

Well, maybe, but the innovators of the new approaches seem lukewarm to a single, rather simple explanation. "Basically, Charles is saying that every time a person looks at a trauma in a safe environment, the stress is reduced," says Frank Gerbode, the inventor of TIR. "I'm not enthralled. Theoretically, Figley's hypothesis means that you could cure PTSD by putting somebody on an anti-anxiety drug [which you can't]. Besides, continuing therapeutic support. Still, the other demonstrators then wondered if perhaps they shouldn't have "turned down" some clients, as well.

If the EMDR contingent aroused the most heart-burnings because of their alleged cherry-picking, they were also the most dismayed by the project's heterodoxy. They objected to the inadequate diagnostic guidelines ("most of the clients didn't even have PTSD," says Shapiro) or clear, systematic protocols; the failure to include more standard (and reputable, one suspects) brief therapies (like flooding or some cognitive-behavioral technique); and the conflation of EMDR which they consider a comprehensive therapy with three treatments targeted more to specific trauma symptoms. "The conception of the project was admirable, the decision to use highly trained clinical demonstrators worthwhile," says Shapiro. "But in the absence of scientific rigor, people will misunderstand the meaning of the outcomes. The field is not going to be swayed by this; few academics, or scientists or sophisticated clinicians will be impressed. The whole thing was a mush."

It is also hard to escape the impression that Shapiro finds it maddening to see her method cast once again into the netherworld of unrecognized, unorthodox, largely untested and unpublished clinical arrivistes who have barely started up the hard trail to official legitimacy. Shapiro has spent eight years of unrelenting effort trying to wrestle EMDR into the family of standard professional and scientific psychology, pushing more strenuously for empirical research than any other mental-health-care innovator in recent history (outside the pharmaceutical industry). She has provided free EMDR training to researchers and trained more than 18,000 clinicians in her approach, which has been the subject of at least 60 clinical research studies. Still, the waves she has made in the field with her outre method and the resistance she has encountered has not particularly surprised her. "It's just what [science philosopher] Thomas Kuhn says," she remarks with resignation. "The old guard has to die off before new paradigms are finally accepted."

In all, what with dropouts, disqualifications and failures to come in for follow-up, the actual number of participants assigned to each approach ranged from 6 to 15 (EMDR 6, TIR and V/KD 9, TFT 15) who actually made it through the entire process. The average time required to achieve results by each method ranged from a high of 254 minutes (TIR, which requires the clients to talk more) to a low of 63 minutes for TFT. The V/KD technique, involving a somewhat extended visualization process, took 113 minutes to complete.

EMDR demonstrators said they had used more time (an average of 172 minutes) than they really needed simply to relieve symptoms, because they felt obliged for ethical reasons to try and do what they normally did go through an elaborate eight-phase treatment protocol. This allowed them to get to know and prepare the client, decide on target events, treat both the target issue and anything else that came up and provide for closure and reevaluation.

If it had been a horse race, which the investigators as well as the innovators were all at pains to deny, the TFT contingent would have won, hands down. Requiring virtually nothing in the way of personal interaction, TFT can bypass all that tedious therapeutic business of joining, empathy, history-taking, reprocessing and the like, and zero in on the problem immediately at hand. With 10-minute treatments not at all unusual (comparatively long, actually), Roger and Joanne Callahan both finished the test early, so to speak, even though they said they were the last ones assigned clients and got the "dregs, including several patients whom other therapists could not help, even one psychotic." Still, says Roger Callahan, "We didn't have enough people, and could have taken a lot more, so we just spent a lot of time chatting [with clients]." They might have produced even more impressive results, he continues, "but we only went in at a third of our power. We understood the treatments we showed were supposed to be those that the average [para- or non-professional] person could do. Afterward, we heard that the others ignored this, and went in with their best shot. We had much more powerful recipes we could have brought to do even better."

When Carbonell and Figley began what they called their "star search," they wanted to get talented but unsung newcomers out of the straw hat circuit and bring them to Broadway. Once the innovators had demonstrated their stuff before a tougher audience than the usual workshop crowd, the investigators hoped to learn more about trauma, stimulate further research and, finally, perhaps uncover some sort of "active ingredient" or powerful antidote to PTSD common to all four approaches. The possibility of achieving any of these goals would have evaporated, of any therapist worth his or her salt produces hypostress during a session." V/KD practitioner Maryanne Reese believes that there are more likely many active ingredients involved, rather than just one. "We don't believe the hypostress-hyper-stress hypothesis is the active ingredient," says Joanne Callahan of TFT. "All the old methods get people to focus on the trauma, and they don't work. We think the new approaches are dealing with the body's underlying energy systems." To Francine Shapiro, Figley's explanation radically oversimplifies EMDR in which she believes the eye movements and the reduction of traumatic symptoms are only part of a more comprehensive cognitive and emotional restructuring. "EMDR is not just a technique that just gets rid of a certain amount of disturbance," says Shapiro. "We try to get in as many changes as possible awareness, insight, new goals for the future."

Carbonell and Figley plan to carry on their project, showcasing both the famous and the obscure among brief approaches to PTSD. Solution-focused and narrative therapies are next on the agenda, and so is something called the Tapas Acupressure Technique (TAT). Developed by Tapas Fleming, an acupuncturist with a background in yoga and Taoism, TAT involves placing two fingers at either side of the nose between the eyes and the other hand firmly against the base of the skull while thinking about the trauma. Publicized via the Internet Trauma Forum, the method was tried by several therapists, who liked it. The opinion among those Figley polled was on the order of, "Well, it's no wackier than TFT, so why not try it?"

Notwithstanding the noisy opposition to EMDR, and probably, soon, the other three therapies given new visibility by their inclusion in this study, the response to Figley and Carbonell's research seems more bemused fascination than outright hostility like watching somebody cross Niagara Falls on a tightrope in a thunderstorm. One colleague recently told Figley, "Well, Charles, I would laugh at anyone else doing this, but you may just have a shot at it." Conservative peers are occasionally a bit more blunt with Carbonell one psychologist asked her if she and Figley "had any validated research to back up that crap you're studying." Carbonell responded by asking him if he had any validated research to back up his own habit of one-hour-a-week talk therapy. The cautious response may suggest the fugitive hope, particularly at a time when the economic Zeitgeist demands ever shorter therapies, that there might just be something to this new, new wave. The promise of brief, cheap, effective treatments to dangle in front of the eyes of managed care executives is strong incentive for open-mindedness.

And yet there are good grounds for being cautious besides the ambiguities of the project itself one being a decent regard for psychotherapy's checkered history. Jay Efran remembers the appearance some years ago of a new psychotherapy approach it doesn't matter which one, the story is legion that showed extraordinary promise. Therapists who used the method, which was amazingly simple, reported clients making faster gains than they had after years of more conventional treatment. There were testimonials and case histories of miraculous turnarounds; followers flocked to weekend trainings, newsletters sprang up, a book or two were published. But then it was found that for certain difficult cases, the method required longer time to work and more integration with standard practices. Eventually, most people who received the new treatment were found to be "chronic," with "deep-seated" issues or attitudes not amenable to speedy cures. In the end, says Efran, the method became largely indistinguishable from any other therapy modality, where it putters on to this day. Says Efran, "We could pull together a whole string of these things, which, as they become known, show themselves to be little different from the ones that went before." On the other hand, Efran is not immune to hope, either, "I still can't resist being intrigued," he says. "What if I paid no attention to something like TFT and it turned out that it worked? I wouldn't want to miss it."

What worries some therapists more than the scientific issues, however, is the possibility that by emphasizing the quick, symptomatic fix, the field is in danger of forgetting that trauma never happens exclusively inside the individual. It is inextricably embedded in a family and social context, and inevitably raises moral and spiritual questions about the whole meaning and purpose of life. "Therapists feel great urgency to provide immediate symptom relief to people in pain," says Washington, D.C., therapist Jeffrey Jay, "but if they don't also address the client's question, 'Why did this happen to me?' they ignore a critical part of his or her suffering, which is about meaning, that requires us to look at the religious and moral community in which the trauma occurred."

In the experience of some trauma therapists, PTSD cannot be adequately treated without addressing broader social, political and spiritual issues, as well as the individual psychological suffering and neurophysiologically based stress reactions. "The trauma of Vietnam vets was not just about killing or experiencing the fear of being killed, it was about an unpopular war and coming home to a country that didn't support them," says trauma therapist Mary Jo Barrett, director of training and consultation at the Center for Contextual Change in Skokie, Illinois. Similarly, Barrett argues, the trauma of childhood sexual abuse is bound up with strong moral and religious taboos about sex and a social climate in which the child's fear of telling is matched by the unwillingness of adults to listen. Barrett, who treats both sexual abuse victims and perpetrators, combines individual and family therapy, encouraging clients to write stories or poetry, as well as renew their spiritual resources. Perpetrators are required to do community service help other offenders, give talks to victims' groups, engage in political work against sexism and racism.

Still, therapists yearn for something that will at least break the impasse that keeps people with PTSD too overwhelmed by their symptoms to even begin engaging in therapy. Trauma therapists report trying the new methods only because near-despair overcame skepticism. "I had no confidence EMDR would work," says Nanci Barthel, a therapist with an agency in Oklahoma City who took free EMDR training offered in the wake of the 1995 bombing. "But I was at the point that I didn't think I wanted to be a therapist anymore. I had such severe caseloads, with so much trauma, and I felt so ineffective." Both EMDR and TIR, which she also learned, changed her life, she says, vastly improving her therapy results. "I can help people move beyond mere survival to improve the quality of their lives they are not just managing the trauma, they have moved beyond it." Kate Sorensen, the therapist who found work on a Navajo reservation so dispiriting she nearly left therapy several years ago, has also seen her practice reborn after learning all four new methods. "These approaches have changed both my work and my life. Getting in touch with people's suffering when I can help them is a thrill. It's the difference between burnout and joy."

These reports, heard over and over, sound like stories of conversion and salvation first I was lost, then I was found that have been too easy for skeptics to dismiss as so much pseudo-religious hot air. Clearly, something "real" is happening to simply reject out of hand the experiences of hundreds of thousands of clients and therapists because empirical trials are lacking seems perverse but what, exactly, is happening isn't so obvious. Perhaps the four approaches will indeed prove to be avatars of a continuously prophesied "new paradigm" in therapy (though Frank Gerbode argues that the field doesn't yet have a commonly agreed upon old paradigm), transforming theory and practice.

But whether or not the "power therapies" will still be around in five years, let alone revolutionize the entire psychotherapeutic worldview, the glowing reports suggest they provide something critical to the practice of therapy: they instill in therapists a sense of confidence and mastery in their own capacity to help people, a feeling of hope that even presumably "hopeless" clients can recover, which is perhaps their most important tool. "I always felt these [traumatized and severely disturbed] clients were unreachable, untouchable, that I wasn't able to address their problems," says Barthel. "But when I took these trainings, I found myself staring hope right in the face hope, which I had never had before, that there are ways to resolve these problems."

Healers must believe in themselves and their therapy, writes Harvard medical anthropologist Arthur Kleinman, in order to stimulate feelings of belief and hope in their clients. This benign mutual collusion in belief and hope, a kind of healing covenant between doctor and patient, therapist and client, is the source of the so-called placebo affect a powerful curative agent in its own right (an estimated 10 to 90 percent improvement rate for medical conditions are due to placebo) that has been wrongly dismissed as an annoying epiphenomenon, a kind of ugly stepsister to "real" treatment, in both physical and mental health care. Certainly, the innovators are unsurprisingly loath to see the word placebo coupled with their own methods, because it connotes something inert, innocuous, accidental, unreal. Roger Callahan even maintains that because TFT arouses so much skepticism in clients, it doesn't get its fair share of placebo cures thus he vouches for its "real" efficacy. And yet, therapists who insist upon their prior skepticism about a new method, and then try it anyway, are more hopeful than skeptical from the beginning, as are the clients who give their assent. Indeed, the toughest-minded skeptic is skeptical about skepticism itself. At heart, all clients and therapists must share some flutterings of hope, even if secret and unadmitted, before embarking together on something new. This willingness to try something new, again and again, this refusal to be beaten down by misery and despair is, finally, the most important "active ingredient" of any therapy.

Mary Sykes Wylie, Ph.D. is Senior Editor of The Family Therapy Networker.

# A Qualitative Study Of Client Perceptions Of TIR:
# A Brief Trauma Treatment
## By Pamela Vest Valentine, Ph.D.

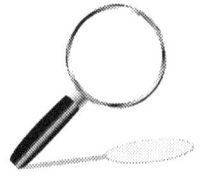

*Crisis Intervention*, 1998, Vol. 4, pp. 1 - 12

PAMELA VEST VALENTINE
Assistant Professor, Social Work Program, University of Alabama at Birmingham

THOMAS EDWARD SMITH
Professor in Social Work at Florida State University. Send requests for reprints to Pamela Valentine, at the University of Alabama at Birmingham, 339 Ullman Bldg. 1212 University Blvd., Birmingham, AL 35294-3350

The purpose of this study was to explore client evaluations of a brief trauma treatment, Traumatic Incident Reduction (TIR). Sixteen clients from four states were interviewed on their experience of TIR using a qualitative research protocol. The practitioners were experienced in TIR and its use in brief therapy. Six domains emerged from an analysis of the transcripts of the interviews: Support, Safety, Structure, Heightened Physiological State, Insight, and End Point. The domains tend to support the principal claims made by proponents of TIR but also add another dimension that has not been previously discussed. Implications of this study for social work practice in crisis counseling, education, and research are discussed.

KEY WORDS: Traumatic Incident Reduction, trauma, brief treatment, qualitative research, ethnography, empowerment

# INTRODUCTION

The population affected by posttraumatic stress disorder (PTSD) is continually growing (Ursano & Fullerton, 1990). Concomitant with PTSD are disorders like substance abuse and depression (Keane & Wolfe, 1990). The effects of PTSD bear on individual stability, interpersonal relationships (Maltz, 1988) and productivity in employment, thus impacting the economy as well as bearing on victims' personal lives. The degree of success in resolving the trauma of victimization has systemic implications. Therefore, identifying effective, brief trauma treatments and systematically evaluating them is a relevant and vital mission for social work. The purpose of this paper is to report on clients' evaluations of one such brief trauma model.

Increasingly, social workers are calling for systematic assessment of clinical practice (Fischer, 1993). As we seek to elevate our professional status, we are increasingly aware that systematic practice evaluation is, central to that process. The motto "Do no harm "links practice evaluation with ethical practice. Finally, both the breadth of client populations and the severity of crisis situations seen by social workers demand implementation of highly effective techniques across diverse settings.

Constraints to practice evaluation have been cited in the literature (Fischer, 1973; Wood, 1982). One of the problems associated with practice evaluation is the assumption that research will be limited to positivist methodology. With positivist methodology, the researcher often measures one reality, assumes linear causality, and demands careful measurement with the goal of reaching statistical significance. Fischer (1993) wrote that practitioners find positivistic research to be highly rigorous and largely irrelevant. Besides disappointment in intense efforts that produce marginally relevant information, practitioners are concerned that rigorous research compromises treatment integrity.

Videka-Sherman (1988) suggests that social workers engage in the best possible research given the constraints of their practice setting. Videka-Sherman writes that the demand for methodological purity discourages practitioners from-engaging in any research. In this study, we sought to evaluate Traumatic Incident Reduction (TIR), a brief trauma intervention, using qualitative methods. In planning and implementing the qualitative research methods, we sought to avoid the rigid demands imposed by rigorous quantitative methods and practitioners' concerns about compromised treatment integrity that can easily result from fitting the intervention to the constraints of the research method.

## Traumatic Incident Reduction

Traumatic Incident Reduction (TIR) (Gerbode, 1989) is a client-respectful, therapist-directed, memory-based therapeutic intervention most similar to imaginal flooding. It is designed to reduce the troublesome symptoms often experienced by survivors of traumatic events. It has been used primarily on verbal adults who are stable enough to focus on a troubling event for a sustained period of time. Traumatic events on which TIR has been used include natural disaster, violence of a non-interpersonal nature like illness, death, and accidents, and interpersonal violence like assault, verbal abuse, incest and rape. Additionally, TIR has been used on both single incident events such as an accident, and on repeated incident events like sexual abuse (Bisbey, 1994; Coughlin, 1995; Valentine, 1995).

TIR stands apart from other practice models in its structure and open-ended length of session. Typically, a session may last three to four hours after which clients will experience a significant sense of relief in their symptoms. The course of TIR depends on the number of traumas that the clients experienced. Thus, there is no typical course of treatment although it is entirely possible that clients who present with a single trauma will terminate after one or two sessions. TIR is structured so that the client and practitioner have distinct, explicated roles. The client makes decisions regarding which traumatic event to review, where to start with the review, on what to focus and how to interpret the event. The practitioner limits remarks to the following:

- when was the event;
- how long did it last;
- go to the beginning of the event and tell me when you are there;
- Review the event silently in your mind and tell me when you are finished;
- tell me what happened.

After the client relates the event as they saw or experienced it, the practitioner begins the cycle of questions again without making empathic nor interpretative remarks. The practitioner terminates the session when she/he detem1ines that the client has resolved the incident for himself/herself.

## Theory Underlying TIR

Originators of TIR pose that its series of structured questions allows clients to focus on the event, to reengage emotionally with the event, and to come to view the event in a different light (Gerbode, 1989). In so doing, the client becomes unencumbered by the event. Several theories support the idea that focus, emotional engagement and cognitive restructuring are components of effective trauma treatment (i.e., cognitive-behavioral, cathartic, & psychoanalytic). Behavioral theory explains that the maintenance of PTSD symptoms is a matter of simple or complex conditioning (Fairband & Brown, 1987). Cognitive theorists believe that old constructs are shattered by the forceful experience of a traumatic event (Janoff-Bulman, 1992). Moore (1993) postulates that for an event to provoke a significant stress reaction (Ellis, 1962), the event must trigger and threaten an aspect of a preexisting belief system (Koss & Burkhart, 1989).. Since the first line of defense is reflexive (Waites, 1993), "insight is a luxury that the mind cannot afford when locked in a struggle for survival" (Everstine & Everstine, 1993, p. 18). The victim begins operating from hastily made constructs, those formed during or immediately after the traumatic incident. While those constructs were relevant to a life-threatening situation, they are not appropriate for everyday living. Yet the new construct is not easily abandoned since it was derived during a heightened physiological response.

Cathartic theorists propose that one must reexperience the heightened physiological state associated with the trauma in order to reevaluate and alter the cognitive distortions that began with the trauma. Cathartic psychotherapies involve strong emotional expression. . Yet arousal alone is not sufficient (Straton, 1990). The client must develop a new perception or redecision of his or her traumatic episode. Often the new perception involves focusing on the decisions made at the time of the traumatic episode. An example of such decisions might be "This will never happen to me again." The redecision is "I can't control whether a similar trauma will happen to me again. I survived it once and I can survive it again." This is similar to the insight sought in psychoanalysis.

TIR presents clients with the opportunity to correct cognitive distortions. Clients retell their story, relive the event in a safe, controlled environment, reexamine the conclusions that were drawn from the experience, and come to a different understanding of the event.

# METHODS

## Overview of Design

The use of ethnoscience guided the methodology in this study. Ethnoscience is based on the assumption that one can describe what people think by analyzing what they say (Fetterman, 1989). Rather than relying upon behavioral observation, ethnoscience analyzes syntactical and semantic relationship among words (e.g., Sells, Smith, Coe, Yoshioka, & Robbins, 1994; Sells, Smith & Sprenkle, 1995). The methodology combined elements from Spradley's (1979, 1980) Developmental Research Sequence (DRS), constant comparative analysis (Glaser & Strauss, 1967; Strauss & Corbin, 1990) and content analysis.

Based on the underpinnings of ethnoscience, exit interviews were conducted with clients who had completed at least one session of TIR. The interviews were tape-recorded, transcribed, and analyzed using domain analysis (Spradley, 1980). Domain analysis requires that researchers examine transcripts of interviews and code them according to a set of semantic relationships that Spradley devised. Because the coding process requires an iterative process in which subsequent transcripts of interviews are coded using domains established in previous transcripts, domain analysis represents an ever-evolving data analytic procedure. Domain analysis has many similarities to constant comparative analysis described by Corbin and Strauss (1990). All but four clients were interviewed by someone other than their primary therapists. Two possible advantages exist in having the interviewer be someone other than the primary therapist: (1) Clients are freed from a fear of offending their therapists, and (2) clients may more readily disclose opinions (i.e., Sells, Smith, & Moon, 1996). In the four cases in which the primary therapist interviewed her own client, we reviewed the transcripts to ascertain whether the depth or breadth of disclosure was similar to those interviews in which someone other than the primary therapist interviewed clients. All interviewers, whether they were primary therapists or not, were experienced in conducting qualitative interviews and had previously participated in ethnographic studies.

## Sample Selection

A total of 16 clients were interviewed. The pool of clients came from Maryland, Michigan, California and Florida. The sampling frame was developed by Metapsychology, an organization founded by Frank Gerbode who founded TIR. Metapsychology provided names and addresses of two TIR-trained therapists who regularly implemented TIR in their work with clients and who might be willing to have their clients interviewed and included in the study. Permission was obtained from these two therapists, their clients, and the primary author's clients. Because this study is exploratory in nature, the opportunistic sampling strategy (Honigman, 1970) was appropriate; furthermore, generalization of study results was not the research goal. Our goal was to understand the dynamics of TIR from clients' perspectives, allowing us to better explicate its theoretical foundations. Of the 16 clients, twelve were women and four were men. Their ages ranged from 21 to 65, with a median age of 33. Fifteen were Caucasian, and one was Asian. All had at least a high school diploma, but not all were employed.

## Types of Traumatic Events Represented in the Sample

Trauma is defined as "an emotional wound or shock that creates substantial, lasting damage to the psychological development of a person." (The American Heritage Dictionary, 1992). TIR gives a client freedom to call traumatic that which he or she experienced as traumatic. Because trauma was defined by clients and not by existing guidebooks, diagnostic criteria for Post-traumatic Stress Disorder listed in the Diagnostic and Statistical Manual (American Psychiatric Association, 1994) were not used to exclude clients. The traumas reported by clients are as follows: abortion (2); molestation by stepfather (3); molestation by brother (1); molestation by baby sitter (1); death of a parent and/or long term illness, followed by death (3); child abuse (1); rape (2); childhood poverty (1); fire (1); car accident (2); and trauma resulting from having been misunderstood by a therapist and forced into a psychiatric hospital (1). Clients' presenting problems included: loss of memory, inability to sleep, inability to concentrate, hyper-anxiety, depression, panic attacks, rage in the context of intimate relationships, temporary inability to tell time, intrusive thoughts, nightmares, confusion, crying, numbness, health problems, stress, feeling dysfunctional, shame, desperation, alcoholism and feeling encumbered by the event.

## Description of the setting

The counseling setting varied by counselor. The primary authors' clients were seen by a social work doctoral student who saw clients in a university-based marriage and family therapy clinic.

Besides providing therapists with supervision of marital and family therapy, the clinic also specialized in trauma work. Typically, the clinic's clients were uninsured and either unemployed or underemployed. Because services were affordable, the clinic received referrals from throughout the city and county.

The other three practice settings differed widely from the university-based marriage and family therapy clinic. Clients were either seen in a private practice setting or, in one case, in the client's home. Of the two practitioners involved in these three sites, one had her MSW and the other practitioner had a high school diploma. Although the educational background of the providers differed greatly, all practitioners in the study were certified in TIR.

Clients' demographics revealed that clients seen in Maryland, Michigan, and California were of a higher socio-economic class than those seen in Florida. For example, one client purchased airfare for his/her therapist to travel from the East Coast to the Midwest where the client lived. Upon arrival, the therapist devoted the better part of a day to provide an intensive TIR session.

## Iterative Domains

The interview protocol had two stages. In the first phase, clients were asked an open-ended question like, "If you were to describe to a friend the process of TIR ... what it was like to go through a session of TIR ... what would you tell the friend?" From there, the interviewer limited his/her remarks to those of clarification and asking for amplification.

The second phase of questions came from themes presented in the open-ended question. To keep the questions as non-leading as possible, iterative questions often began with, "Some people have said that…" The client was asked if they could comment on whether that aspect of TIR was true for them. Other questions had clauses like, "What, if anything, do you have to say about…?"

In both phases, clients were introduced to the interview protocol with the following paragraph:

> What we are interested in is your opinion. We want to know what the process was like for you. We want you to recount your experience. . . not the traumatic story. . . but what it was like for you from when you first began TIR to when it was over. This is not a test; we only care about what you think. It will help us do a better job in the future and/or it will help future therapists and clients know the strengths and weaknesses of this procedure. Do you have any questions?

# RESULTS

Following a domain analysis, six domains emerged: Support, Safety, Structure, Heightened Physiological State, Insight, and End Point. In Table 1, each domain is listed, together with subdomains and included terms. The included terms on the right-hand side of the table are direct quotations taken from clients. The middle column represents domains that initially emerged from the analysis and the left column represents the domains into which the sub domains were clustered. Within the first domain, clients believed that support from their therapists' use of TIR came from: Listening and Nonverbal Communication of Empathy. Interestingly, clients' portrayed therapists as listening intently and being extraordinarily patient. Clients did not consider therapists' avoidance of overt praise as harming the therapeutic relationship. If anything, the ability to patiently hear the same story repeatedly was noted as a significant feature of the listening abilities of TIR therapists.

| **Support** | Listening | • Someone willing to sit with you and listen to you tell the same story 25 times.<br>• Not trying to please you |
| | Nonverbal communication of empathy | • The pats-on-the-back are missing; I don't know if that is good or bad.<br>• I know she is 'interested in what I am saying<br>• Body language<br>• Acknowledges what I say |
| **Safety** | Comfortable with therapist | • It is important to trust the other person<br>• I don't know if you have to like the therapist, but you have to feel safe with her. |
| | Non-evaluative/ no teaching | • *They do no interpreting; and they let you interpret<br>• No judgments, therefore I control it.<br>• My version of the story is THE version<br>• I won't be made to feel wrong<br>• The less the facilitator inputs, the better |
| | Unlimited time | • Listens to you for as long as it takes |

| Structure | Preparation | • Be rested, fed, and safe.<br>• Explained what would happen, what kind of questions would be asked. |
|---|---|---|
| | Focus | • Focused on the problem, not on the facilitator *I confronted what I avoid<br>• It isolates the event<br>• Pulls me back on focus<br>• The structure kept me feeling safe. |
| | Rote predictability | • Procedure controls flooding of memories<br>• It creates boundaries |
| | Roles | • I'm in control; it put me in the driver's seat<br>• The therapist guides me without being controlling<br>• We worked on MY agenda<br>• Makes it safe<br>• The client does the work.<br>• It's up to you (client) |
| | Repetition | • You start to go into more detail; you can't stay out side the event any longer.<br>• Helped work it through my body, head, and soul.<br>• Thinking through the event becomes a mental map.<br>• Repetition helps reexperience it<br>• Your senses are involved<br>• Remember more details; I saw more of what happened. |
| **Heightened Physiological State** | Somatic symptoms | • Crying<br>• Wanting to throw up<br>• Headache<br>• Lump in my throat<br>• Pain in my chest |

| | Intense emotions | • The pain tells you something real happened<br><br>• I started to shake inside<br>• You have to view the event to feel the pain.<br>• Indignation<br>• Vulnerable<br>• Disbelief<br>• It was like "therapy concentrate"<br>• Got in touch with a part of me |
|---|---|---|
| **Insight** | Problem identified | • I realized I was doing something that caused me difficulty.<br>• Themes in regular therapy surfaced<br>• It put the problem in perspective<br>• Cleaned up the event for me |
| | Self validation | • Memories are true even though you' have no one to confirm it<br>• It wasn't my fault |
| | Decision at time of event | • I won't be rear-ended again. |
| **End Point** | Saturation point | • You start getting detached, bored; it is time to let it go.<br>• Breeze through the story, leaving out details.<br>• Unimportant parts lose their power<br>• Good to . . . make myself live through it again so that it becomes mundane. |
| | Drained | • I might feel drained, but I feel more at ease |
| | Peace | |
| | | • I felt grounded, comforted |
| | Relief | |
| | | • Like passing a kidney stone<br>• Negative emotions never come back af- |

| | Empowered | ter the session.<br><br>• It IS possible to heal from this.<br>• Stronger; I survived<br>• Liberated . . .not having to see a therapist now<br>• Restored potential<br>• Before I was passive and controlled by the incident; now I've gained control<br>• I' ve had more energy since then |
|---|---|---|
| | Diminished symptoms | • Felt less pain at the end<br>• My avoidance of ambulances was gone<br>• Less afraid of the experience |

TABLE 1: Six domains of TIR

The second domain, Safety, included three subdomains: Comfortable with Therapist, Non-Evaluative/No Teaching, and Unlimited Time. The first sub domain was not surprising. Clients put a premium on being able to relax with and trust their therapist. The second subdomain, Non-Evaluative/No Teaching was less intuitive. Therapists' insistence that they not interpret clients' stories enabled clients to feel that their stories were credible, and more importantly, that were not being evaluated by therapists. Clients were emphatic that less input by therapists was preferable; this gave clients a sense of control over their narratives that had been previously missing. This was consistent with the belief that the sense of unlimited time was critical to allow clients to explore and unfold their narratives. Both the sense of Non-Evaluation and the Unlimited Time were critical in providing clients a sense of safety in TIR.

The third domain, Structure, had five subdomains: Preparation, Focus, Rote Predictability, Roles, and Repetition. Clients believed that the first subdomain was important in preparing them for the rigors of TIR. Because recall of trauma can be intense, overtly preparing clients for the experience decreased the shock of the memories and allowed clients to become increasingly desensitized to them. The second subdomain, .

Focus, was cited by clients as important to keep attention on the problem and not on the facilitator (i.e., therapist). Keeping focused on the problem allowed clients to confront what they normally avoided, isolated the event and finally increased the sense of safety. The third subdomain, Rote Predictability, complemented the first two subdomains. Clients believed that the predictability established boundaries; this was especially important since recall of traumatic memories was painful and threatened to emotionally overwhelm clients. The fourth subdomain, Roles, echoed many of the themes heard in the second domain: client control, safety, emphasizing client initiative, and de-emphasizing therapeutic interpretation. In the fifth and last sub domain, Repetition, clients expounded on the value of countlessly repeating the story of the traumatic event. Included among the benefits were that the recalled memories became richer in detail, clients were able to create a mental map of what happened and who was responsible, and clients experienced peace of mind by finally being able to confront images that they had been previously unable to do.

The fourth domain, Heightened Physiological State, had two subdomains: Somatic Symptoms and Intense Emotions. The somatic symptoms were those experienced by clients as they recalled the traumatic events. It included crying, sensations of nausea, headaches, and chest pains. For many clients, these somatic symptoms confirmed the veracity of the recalled events. The second subdomain, intense emotions, was summed up by one client who called TIR a "therapy concentrate." The intensity of the emotions allowed a sense of indignation, disbelief, vulnerability and pain to come forward. For many of these clients, these intense emotions, previously attributed to other factors, now were placed in perspective. Clients were able to understand the depth of their emotions regarding their past trauma; for many of them, this new understanding represented a source of intense relief.

The fifth domain was Insight. Insight refers to the cognitive explanation that clients' mental maps were altered at the time of the traumas and that TIR facilitated clients' reexamining how those maps were altered. The three subdomains were: Problem Identification, Self Validation, and Decision at Time of Event. Problem identification refers to the client's being able to understand what the problem was and ways in which they contributed to the problem. Furthermore, clients felt that TIR allowed them to put the problem in a new context, to connect it to themes with which they had dealt in prior therapy session, and/or to "put the problem in perspective." The second subdomain, Self Validation, points to the clients' realizing that memories are true, even though one has no external source to confirm the memory. This subdomain relates to the Heightened Physiological State, mentioned above because the shear depth of emotion felt upon recall of the event convinced the clients that the event was real. Other clients expressed relief in realizing that they were not at fault in the traumatic incident. The third and final subdomain, Decision at the Time of the Event, speaks to the client's insight into how his/her mental map was altered at the time of the event. After realizing that a decision was made, the client can choose for herself/himself whether that decision is still appropriate after the event. An example of a decision was, "I won't be rear-ended again." Should clients realize that they made an intention over which they have no control, they may abandon that intention and place their efforts in areas over which they have more control.

The sixth and final domain, End Point, had six subdomains: Saturation Point, Drained, Peace, Relief, Empowered, and Diminished Symptoms. The saturation point involves indicators that the story has been told a sufficient number of times and that telling the story feels less troublesome. Boredom with the story, ease of telling the story, deletion of details, loss of interest in the unimportant parts, and a sense of the mundane were the indicators of saturation point. The second subdomain, Drained, pointed to the physical sensation felt after having been highly aroused in the reliving of the event. We noted the Florida clients expressed this feeling with more regularity than clients from other regions of the country. Since the clients' experience of TIR seemed consistent across the locations, one explanation for this variation is that the Florida clients who were from lower socio-economic structure, were newer to therapy in general and less accustomed to confronting harsh psychological realities. Of interest is that while some clients said that they were drained, they also said that they felt more at ease. The third sub domain, Peace, was derived from statements like, "I feel grounded," or "I feel comforted." Relief, the fourth sub domain, further reflects the comforted feeling clients had. As one client put it, "It was like passing a kidney stone." Another, who had undergone TIR for various events said that the negative emotions associated with the event prior to TIR never came back after the session. The fifth subdomain, Empowered, came from clients using words like "stronger, liberated, restored potential, gaining control and increased energy." Just knowing that they faced the event and survived it meant that they felt stronger. One noted that he/she moved from passivity to taking control. Incidentally, the liberated statement was in reference to not having to see a therapist any longer! The sixth and final domain, Diminished Symptoms, dealt with the decrease in the sense of pain and fear surrounding the event. One client spoke specifically of his /her presenting problem, avoidance of ambulances, noting that immediately after the TIR session, this problem was gone.

# DISCUSSION

In this study, 16 clients from four states were interviewed on their experience of TIR using a qualitative research protocol. The practitioners were experienced in TIR and its use in brief therapy. Six domains emerged from an analysis of the transcripts of the interviews: Support, Safety, Structure, Heightened Physiological State, Insight, and End Point. The domains tend to support the principal claims made by proponents of TIR but also add another dimension that has not been previously discussed. Clients in this sample believed strongly that the use of TIR empowered them to make decisions and to develop their self-confidence in a way that ordinary psychotherapy had failed to do. Overall, the findings have a number of implications for social work practice, education, and research.

## Implications for Social Work Practice

Social work practitioners are being confronted daily with clients who have experienced both interpersonal and disaster-related trauma. Because such experiences are frequently disorienting and devastating, trauma treatment is especially challenging. Managed care presents additional challenges like limiting the number of sessions and insisting upon one hour sessions. This combination suggests that traditional psychotherapeutic approaches may not be adequate. Clients' reactions in this study suggest that TIR represents a viable brief therapy modality that is consistent with many social work values like empowerment and self-determination.

## Implications for Social Work Research

The use of qualitative methodologies are increasingly being used to study brief and innovative therapies (e.g., Sells et al., 1994; Sells et al., 1996; Smith, Jenkins, & Sells, 1995). Although use of these methodologies can be exacting, they provide a valuable method to discover relationships among textual data that would otherwise not be possible. Qualitative research can best be seen as a complement to quantitative research methods (Sells, et al., 1995). Because qualitative research methods help form hypotheses and suggest avenues of research, they become essential tools in planning quantitative confirmatory studies. For example, in this study, empowerment was suggested by clients as a key advantage of TIR. This had not been cited previously by TIR's proponents. Its endorsement by clients suggests that future quantitative studies of TIR should include a measure of empowerment as well as the traditional measures of PTSD and depression.

# CONCLUSIONS

The findings from this study provide support for the belief that Traumatic Incident Reduction can remediate symptomatology that arise from interpersonal violence and disaster-related trauma, and is a viable approach to time-limited treatment. Because this study used a convenience sample that cannot be generalized to all clients or even to all TIR clients, any conclusions at this time are modest. Nonetheless, the clients provided an encouraging endorsement of the claims made by TIR's proponents. In fact, the sense of empowerment experienced by clients was a notable addition to benefits already noted in the literature. It is clear, however, that confirmatory studies are needed if a greater understanding of TIR is to become realized. The lack of studies on TIR's efficacy eventually will undermine the credibility of claims made by its proponents and by clients in this study. A current study is underway in which an outcome study using an experimental design will provide further answers about the credibility of TIR. Clearly, the potential of TIR will remain unfulfilled without efforts to ascertain its efficacy.

## References

American Psychiatric Association. (1994). Diagnostic and statistical manual of mental disorders (4th ed.). Washington, DC: Author.

Bisbey, L. B. (1994). No longer a victim: A treatment outcome study of crime victims with post-traumatic stress disorder. Doctoral dissertation for California School of Professional Psychology, San Diego. University Micro Films International publication number: 952269.

Coughlin, W. E. (1995). Traumatic Incident Reduction: Efficacy in treating anxiety symptomatology. Unpublished doctoral dissertation, Union University.

Ellis, A. (1962). Reason and emotion in psychotherapy. New York: Lyle Stuart.

Everstine, D. and Everstine, L. (1993). The trauma response: Treatment for emotional injury. New York: W. W. Norton & Company.

Fairbank, J. A. and Brown, T. A. (1987). Current behavioral approaches to the treatment of post-traumatic stress disorder. The Behavior Therapist, 5, (1),22-36.

Fetterman, D, M. (1989). Ethnography step by step. Newbury Park, CA: Sage.

Fischer, J. (1993). Empirically-based practice: The end of ideology? Journal of Social Services Research, 18, (112) 19-64.

Fischer, J. (1973). Is casework effective? A review. Social Work, 18, 5-20.

French, G. D. and Gerbode, F. A. (1993). The Traumatic Incident Reduction Workshop (2nd Ed.). Menlo Park: IRM Press.

Gerbode, F. (1989). Beyond psychology: An introduction to metapsychology. Palo Alto: IRM Press.

Gerbode, F. and Moore, R. (1994). Beliefs and intentions in RET. Journal of Rational-Emotive and Cognitive Behavior Therapy, /2, (1),27-45.

Glaser, B. G. and Strauss, A. L. (1967). The discovery of grounded theory: Strategies for qualitative research. New York: Aldine.

Honigman, J. J. (1970). Sampling in ethnographic field work. In R. Haroll & R. Cohen (Eds.)., Hqndbook of research in cultural anthropology. Garden City, NJ: Natural History Press.

Janoff-Bulman, B. (1992). Shattered assumptions. New York: The Free Press. Keane, T. and Wolfe, J. (1990). Comorbidity in post-traumatic stress disorder: An analysis of community and clinical studies. Journal of Applied Social Psychology, 20, (21),1176-1788.

Koss, M. and Burkhart, B. (1989). A conceptual analysis of rape victimization: Long-term effects and implications for treatment. Psychology of Women Quarterly 13, 27-40.

Maltz, W. (1988). Identifying and treating the sexual repercussions of incest: A couples therapy approach. Journal of Sex and Marital Therapy, 14 (9), 142-169.

Moore, R. H. (1993). Cognitive-emotive treatment of the posttraumatic stress disorder. In W. Dryden and L. Hill (Eds.) Innovations in rational-emotive therapy. Newbury Park, CA: Sage Publications.

Sells, S., Smith, T. E., Coe, M. J., Yoshioka, M. and Robbins, J. (1994). An ethnography of couple and therapist experiences in Reflecting Team practice. Journal of Marital and Family Therapy, 20, 247-266

Sells, S. P., Smith, T. E. ,and Moon, S. (1996). An ethnographic study of client and therapist perceptions of therapy effectiveness in a university-based training clinic. Journal of Marital and Family Therapy, 22 (3), 321 342.

Smith, T. E., Jenkins, D. A. and Sells, S. P. (1995). Reflecting Teams: Voices of diversity. Journal of Family Psychotherapy, 6(2), 49-70.

Soukhanov, A. H. (1992). The American heritage dictionary (3rd ed.). Boston: Houghton Mifflin Company. Spradley, J. P. (1979). The ethnographic interview. New York: Holt, Rinehart and Winston.

Spradley, J. P. (1980). Participant observation. New York: Holt, Rinehart and Winston.

Straton, D. (1990). Catharsis reconsidered. Australian and New Zealand Journal of Psychiatry, 24, 543-551. Strauss, A. and Corbin, J. (1990). Basics of qualitative research. Newbury Park, CA: Sage.

Drsano, R. and Fullerton, C. (1990). Cognitive and behavioral responses to trauma. Journal of Applied Psychology, 20, (21), 1766-1775..

Valentine, P. (1995). Traumatic incident reduction: A review of a new intervention. Journal of Family Psychotherapy, 6 (2), 73-78.

Valentine, P. and Smith, T. E. (1995, October). Brief treatment of traumatized clients: An ethnographic study. Paper presented at the annual meeting of the National Association of Social Workers, Philadelphia, PA. Videka-Sherman, L. (1988). Meta-analysis of research on social work practice mental health. Social work, 33, 325-338.

Waites, E. A. (1993). Trauma and survival: Post-traumatic and dissociative disorders in women. New York: W. W. Norton and Co..

Wood, M. (1982). Evaluating practice: Science as faith. Social Casework, 63, 266-272

# 10 Exposure Therapy Renewed

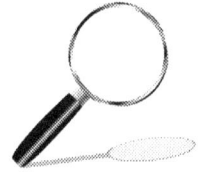

## Phillip M. Massad and Timothy L. Hulsey

Journal of Psychotherapy Integration .Copyright 2006 by the American Psychological Association. 2006, Vol. 16, No. 4, 417–428 1053-0479/06/$12.00 DOI: 10.1037/1053-0479.16.4.417 417. Reproduced with permission.

Recurrence of posttraumatic stress disorder (PTSD) symptoms after treatment has been a long-standing problem. Recent theories of PTSD suggest that different types of processing (i.e., sensory vs. conceptual) may contribute to the return of symptoms. Patients who process their experience primarily via sensory cues (i.e., focusing on the specific environmental cues present at the time of the trauma) are more likely to develop the automatic, physiologically based symptoms of PTSD, which are often the most debilitating. Exposure therapy, based on conditioning principles related to extinction, may be a first-line course of treatment. Contemporary learning theory suggests ways to change exposure treatment to limit the reappearance of symptoms. This research suggests that lengthy and numerous exposure sessions, the use of conditioned inhibitors, and creating a maximal excitatory exposure context can yield efficacious treatment and minimize the likelihood of symptom renewal. Moreover, means for constructing the optimal exposure context are discussed via the use of free association.

Individuals treated for posttraumatic stress disorder (PTSD) often experience a recurrence of symptoms (Breslau, 1998). In what follows, we examine current theory and research on symptom recurrence and suggest ways to reduce the odds of renewal in the treatment of PTSD. Because of their widespread use and empirically demonstrated efficacy, we focus primarily on exposure therapy (ET) and extinction in the treatment of PTSD symptoms.

Phillip M. Massad, Institute of Rural Health, Idaho State University; Timothy L. Hulsey, Department of Psychology, Virginia Commonwealth University.

Correspondence concerning this article should be addressed to Phillip M. Massad, Institute of Rural Health, Idaho State University, Pocatello, ID 83202. E-mail: massphil@isu.edu

ET is a circumscribed procedure that capitalizes on the learning-theory construct of extinction. The assumption is that by exposing patients to feared stimuli in a safe context, their fear responding will diminish. Although ET is often used to treat phobias and fears, it also provides an effective treatment for alleviating the symptoms of PTSD (Paunovic, 1997; Rothbaum & Schwartz, 2002). As such, the findings and recommendations we offer would likely apply equally well to phobias and panic symptoms in addition to those arising from PTSD (Jones & Barlow, 1990).

Recent theoretical and empirical findings support the notion that stimuli may be processed differentially during and/or after a trauma (Brewin & Holmes, 2003; Ehlers & Clark, 2000; Halligan, Clark, & Ehlers, 2002). Although these theories differ in their specifics, they underscore the role of nonconscious, cognitive processes in producing the automatic physiological and behavioral responses that define PTSD (Brewin, Dalgleish, & Joseph, 1996; Ehlers & Clark, 2000). In these models, some individuals experience (and reexperience) their trauma predominantly through perceptual, "data-driven" processing (i.e., attend to the perceptual elements of the trauma such as smell, sounds, etc.). As a result of this emphasis on the perceptual content characterizing the trauma, they tend to deemphasize the elaboration of meaning elements of the trauma (i.e., how does one integrate the experience with previous beliefs?). Therefore, these patients appear more likely to develop the automatic, physiological symptoms (e.g., flashbacks, autonomic hyperarousal, hypervigilance, exaggerated startle response) of PTSD that are often described as the most debilitating (Brewin & Holmes, 2003; Halligan, Michael, Clark, & Ehlers, 2003).

Ostensibly then, different interventions may be required if we are to address effectively the symptoms that arise from this automatic, sensory–perceptual cognitive style versus the more deliberate, verbal– conceptual dichotomy of encoding/elaborating the trauma experiences found in other patients. It seems reasonable to suggest that individuals who primarily manifest data-driven or sensory sequelae to trauma, such as flashbacks, intrusive imagery, and physiological reactions, may be particularly suited to treatment via exposure therapy that emphasizes extinction.[1] Although ET-based treatment of the automatic elements of trauma responding may have value for most all PTSD victims, it may be particularly beneficial for those individuals who predominantly manifest these automatic, physiological symptoms of PTSD.

# EXPOSURE: EXTINCTION AND RENEWAL

Extinction has proven to be an effective method for changing conditioned automatic responding in a variety of disorders (Domjan, 2003). However, because it is very difficult to ensure the complete extinction of the stimulus-response (S-R) connections in the clinical treatment of PTSD, patients treated with exposure therapies will always remain vulnerable to the renewal of

---

[1] Patients who report being overwhelmed by sensory impressions versus those who evince more conceptual processing (e.g., awareness of danger, attributions of responsibility, violations of pretrauma beliefs about self and the world) should be distinguishable by anecdotal accounts. Also, simple scaling and use of a cognitive questionnaire have been used with some success to differentiate data-driven from conceptual processors (Halligan et al., 2003; Murray, Ehlers, & Mayou, 2002).

the previous S-R associations. Clinicians using in vivo or imaginal types of exposure therapies are limited by their inability to exactly replicate the conditions that defined the original traumatic situation. Thus, symptoms may recur when stimuli associated with the original trauma (but not directly and sufficiently addressed in the treatment setting) arise. This renewal of the S-R connections in turn reactivates the automatic trauma responses associated with PTSD.

Renewal has been defined as the recovery of responding following extinction. Renewal is apparently caused by the patient's removal from the extinction context (Domjan, 2003). Patients who develop PTSD may extinguish the original fear response to certain conditioned stimuli in therapy only to have it return (i.e., "renew") in other contexts that more closely resemble those present during the original trauma. This is a critical limitation of exposure or extinction treatments. These treatments do not *eliminate* the underlying associations between the stimuli associated with the trauma (e.g., smells, colors, sounds, etc.) and the danger of the original trauma situation (the unconditioned stimulus, or US). The connections are not forgotten or unlearned. Rather, they remain.[2] Although these connections may be inhibited by new learning, they can always be triggered by environmental cues and reemerge. So, for the clinician, it is imperative that exposure be optimized to ensure that the original learning remains suppressed.

If associations are not unlearned, how then do we understand the reduction of fear responses that accompanies exposure treatment? One popular notion is that contextual cues evident in both the trauma incident (i.e., acquisition) and the exposure therapy (i.e., extinction) settings *disambiguate* the significance of conditioned stimuli (CS; Bouton, 1993, 1994). That is, during the trauma event there is no ambiguity about the meaning of stimuli because the CS (e.g., helicopter noise) signals only one thing: attack (i.e., US delivery). However, when CS (e.g., helicopter noises, gunfire, etc.) are present both during the trauma and exposure, they have an ambiguous meaning. In the original trauma situation (i.e., acquisition), they signal an impending US (e.g., attack), whereas in exposure (i.e., extinction) they might signal the absence of the feared result (Domjan, 2003). Consequently, contextual elements (e.g., temperature, smells, etc.) present during extinction become conditioned inhibitors.[3] They come to predict the absence of the feared traumatic event (US) more effectively than does the CS (e.g., helicopter noise) alone. Thus, a CS present during both acquisition and extinction is more susceptible to contextual interpretation than a CS that has been presented only during acquisition. In this model, renewal occurs because memories of the

---

[2] 2 Spontaneous recovery is a related phenomenon, which, like renewal, shows that extinction does not result in unlearning. Spontaneous recovery involves a partial return to acquisition performance when there has been a delay between the conclusion of extinction and the test phase (i.e., reintroduction to the CS). Renewal, on the other hand, requires no such passage of time to demonstrate that learning or inhibition in one context is not static when the context is changed. Nevertheless, contemporary thinking is that both phenomena are likely tied to changes in the context (i.e., from extinction to the test phase) because the passage of time (i.e., the delay interval in spontaneous recovery) likely involves a change in contextual cues (Domjan, 2003).

[3] 3 Stimuli (i.e., CS–) can signal the absence of a US in the presence of the CS+, which, ordinarily, signals the US presence. Thus, there is inhibitory conditioning of the CS+ because of the CS–.

trauma (i.e., excitatory conditioning) return when the contextual cues that were present during extinction or exposure treatment are not available to inhibit them.

This line of reasoning predicts that renewal would be greatest in contexts that do not resemble those present during the extinction therapy. In other words, the more closely the setting for the exposure treatment resembles the original setting where the fear was acquired, the more effective the treatment is likely to be. In classical conditioning terms, the setting of the original trauma would be considered as Setting A. The setting of the extinction therapy would also be Setting A; hence AA represents these sequential contexts of acquisition and extinction. In this example, let us say a rider falls off his horse at a rodeo in the Houston Astrodome (see Table 1 for possible conditioning sequences). Although the rider may develop a fear of horses (i.e., the CS), he may at the same time develop associations between the trauma of falling and the contextual cues of the arena, such as its size, color of seats, and smell. If the rider chose to get back on the horse, he might do so at the next rodeo held at the Astrodome (i.e., Context A) or at a rodeo to be held at Reliant Stadium (Context B). Such an event could be tantamount to extinction if we assume that the rider will not fall off the horse in this second event. Subsequently, the cowboy might ride in a third event which, in extinction terminology, would constitute the "test phase."

| Acquisition | Extinction | Renewal test | Sequence |
|---|---|---|---|
| Astrodome | Astrodome | Astrodome | AAA |
| Astrodome | Reliant | Astrodome | ABA |
| Astrodome | Astrodome | Reliant | AAB |
| Astrodome | Reliant | Minute Maid | ABC |

Table 1. Conditioning Sequence

In the language of S-R psychology, the AAA sequence (i.e., acquisition, extinction, and test) would yield less renewal than AAB or even an ABA sequence because extinction is dependent on context. Reexperiencing the feared situation in the same context but with a different outcome is more likely to inhibit the original S-R connection than is experiencing the altered outcome in a different context. However, renewal in the AAB and ABA sequences should be equal because each involves a change from the extinction context to a nonextinction one (i.e., from A, the Astrodome, to B, Reliant Stadium, and vice versa). In summary, renewal for AAA < ABA = AAB because generalization of context from B to A should be the same as that from A to B.

Other formulations by Bouton (Bouton, 1993; Bouton & Nelson, 1998) suggest that the inhibition of responding, relative to excitatory conditioning, may have a much steeper generalization decrement across contexts. Hence, we would expect renewal in an ABC series of contexts to be similar to an AAB renewal because both groups would have an equivalent generalization decrement of inhibitory conditioning. Unfortunately these predictions have not been substantiated by recent empirical work. Thomas, Larsen, and Ayres (2003) found that AAB renewal is weaker than ABA renewal and that AAB renewal is weaker than ABC renewal.

So, what does all this mean? The findings of Thomas and colleagues (2003) suggest that our cowboy (let us call him "Bob") will demonstrate fewer renewal phenomena if (a) he gets exposure treatment in the Astrodome (i.e., the same site where he fell off the horse; Context A) rather than in Reliant Stadium (Context B), and (b) he is tested for renewal in Reliant Stadium (Context B; Sequence AAB). Furthermore, Bob should demonstrate fewer renewal responses than Cowboy Walt, who, like Bob, got bucked off in the Astrodome, but in contrast gets exposure treatment in Reliant Stadium (Context B) and then gets tested for renewal in the Astrodome (Context A; Sequence ABA). Contrary to Bouton's predictions (Bouton, 1993; Bouton & Nelson, 1998), the presence of renewal phenomena for the cowboy(s) would be greater in the ABA condition than in the AAB condition and greater in the ABC condition than in the AAB condition. Thomas and colleagues (2003) assert that the ostensible and heretofore unconsidered explanation is *that the effectiveness of a US is determined by how surprising or unexpected it is.*

This is the critical assumption of the Rescorla–Wagner model that has dominated research on classical conditioning since the 1970s (Rescorla & Wagner, 1972). To paraphrase, this model asserts that, during exposure treatment, Cowboy Bob would be more "surprised" by the absence of danger (US) in the Astrodome, where he originally fell, than in Reliant Stadium, where he had never fallen. Accordingly, the explicit CS (e.g., the horse) and contextual stimuli (i.e., aspects of the arena) will lose more associative value as a function of nonreinforcement (i.e., Bob does not get thrown off) in the original stadium, the Astrodome, than if extinction occurred in a new setting, such as Reliant. The upshot is that the more similar the exposure (extinction) context is relative to the context of original acquisition, the more CS excitatory value will be lost and the more effective the treatment is likely to be.[4]

## TREATMENT IMPLICATIONS AND RENEWAL RESEARCH

So what is the clinical utility of this information? The clinical implications of either Bouton's (Bouton, 1993; Bouton & Nelson, 1998) or Thomas and colleagues' (2003) explanations are that the exposure therapy context should be as similar as possible to the original learning context. However, the specific modifications that are likely to maximize the effectiveness of exposure therapy hinge on a careful reading of these findings. To summarize, Bouton's (Bouton, 1993; Bouton & Nelson, 1998) explanations of renewal are that (a) extinction is context driven (inhibition acquired during the extinction phase is lost when the patient shifts from the exposure context to a new context) and (b) although both excitatory and inhibitory generalization decre-

---

[4] 4 This model asserts that if lambda represents the asymptote of learning possible with the US, and V the associative value of the stimuli that precede the US, then the "surprise value" of the US will be lambda − V. Early in conditioning trials, there are substantial increments in associative value of V (i.e., the explicit CS and contextual stimuli), but this associative value increases by smaller increments as the trials proceed. In the case of renewal, failing to reinforce the CS in an excitatory context (i.e., A) will cause it to lose more associative value than a failure to reinforce the same stimulus in a less excitatory context (i.e., B) because the former scenario would be more surprising.

ments occur between extinction and renewal contexts, the inhibitory decrement is greater. Thus, the likelihood of renewal will increase as a function of changes in contextual stimuli between the extinction and renewal contexts. Thomas's version of the renewal phenomenon, on the other hand, asserts that extinction occurs as a result of exposing the patient to the feared CS in an optimally excitatory context to increase the likelihood that the patient will be surprised by the failure of the US to follow the CS.

One obvious implication of the research on reducing renewal and improving the effectiveness of exposure involves careful exploration of the patient's phenomenology to determine in what contexts the patient most expects danger (i.e., in what contexts the patient typically manifests the most fear). In exposure work, the patient is asked to provide detail about the trauma. These elements come to comprise the essential elements of the exposure episodes (Foa & Rothbaum, 2001). Such an exposure architecture relies on the patient's conscious awareness of the details of the original trauma context. However, this method is something like the drunk who looks for his car keys under the lamppost because that is where the light is, not where he last saw his keys. The most debilitating symptoms of PTSD occur as a result of nonconscious, automatic cognitive processes that lie outside of awareness and are not available for recall or discussion (see Brewin & Holmes, 2003).

To elicit a more comprehensive mapping of the US–CS associations that underlie the nonconscious, automatic responding associated with PTSD, we turn to the concept of free association (Freud, 1953). Free association, as developed in psychoanalytic and neoanalytic therapies, attempts to discover associative links in the person's mind by allowing him or her to verbalize thoughts, feelings, and fantasies without restraint (Wolberg, 1988). Empirical studies on this technique show that it does facilitate retrieval of information, both verbal and imagery, that is not available to consciousness (see Bornstein, 1993, for a review).

The elementary principles of classical conditioning maintain that a web of associations and generalization gradients exists for any conditioning event (Dollard & Miller, 1950). To be maximally effective, second- and third-order associations should be used in exposure work. By addressing the complex web of associations linked to the trauma via free association, the clinician may construct, as much as possible, a fuller accounting of the various potential triggers for PTSD responding, particularly when the patient is too anxious to participate more fully in delineating the trauma context (Wilson & Smith, 1968).

We must also realize that many patients may not be able to identify the stimulus complex that leads to automatic responding (Ehlers & Clark, 2000; Loftus, 1993). In these instances, free association affords the possibility of reconstructing those elements of the stimulus complex that lie outside of awareness and thereby develop a more comprehensive exposure scenario. For example, if a rape victim begins by describing the street where the assault began, she might be able to provide details about the pavement (e.g., it was gravel). In a free association format, she might add that she was thrown to the gravel, it cut her knee, and she smelled its musky odor. The exposure context thus revealed will be maximally excitatory and, consistent with Thomas and colleagues' (2003) formulation, will reduce more effectively the renewal of responding triggered by environmental cues.

Exposure across different contexts is also desirable because multiple contexts increase the probability of more anticipated US–CS excitatory connections (Bouton, 1993; Bouton & Nelson, 1998; Thomas et al., 2003). These connections are more fully tempered than those treated by extinction in only one environment, which can never fully replicate contextual features of the original acquisition.[5] Stated differently, multiple contexts provide the best potential of replicating the greatest number of acquisition elements (or stimuli similar to them) and thereby achieve optimal excitatory exposure.

Certain trauma theorists have already capitalized on this idea. The traumatic incident reduction (TIR) approach asks the patient to describe not only the trauma incident that precipitated treatment but all other similar traumas and related events (Figley, 2002). This approach attempts to construct an array of connections to earlier associated incidents. This process may activate memories of important details of the recent trauma that heretofore have been omitted or forgotten. In this way, TIR makes use of verbally mediated generalization gradients, which will broaden the exposure treatment stimuli and thus reduce the likelihood of renewal.

## CONDITIONED INHIBITION AND EXPOSURE

Now, we turn to the second component of extinction, conditioned inhibition. This phenomenon occurs when a stimulus (e.g., police officer) is present and inhibits an outcome that might ordinarily occur otherwise (e.g., taunting between two inebriated Red Sox and Yankee fans). This suppression aspect of extinction is often overlooked in exposure treatment. By attending carefully to the factors that affect conditioned inhibition, stimuli that predict the absence of the threat can be made more explicit. Research has found that renewal of conditioned emotional responses can be countered by presenting cues that were present in the extinction phase (Brooks, Palmatier, Garcia, & Johnson, 1999). For example, stimuli such as color, music, or other sounds might be accentuated in the exposure trials to make them stand out as part of the associative learning event. In clinical practice, we might ask a combat veteran to become aware of his wife's facial features when he relates his story of trauma to her. We might also play soothing music in the background during exposure trials, with the melody signaling the absence of danger (i.e., a CS–) that the veteran could utilize in other situations. He could focus on the feel of his truck's upholstery or the texture of his cat's fur while undergoing exposure and use these stimuli to inhibit renewal of the previous associations in other contexts.

It is worth noting that group exposure therapy offers additional opportunities for inhibitory conditioning, because the members of the group become "conditioned inhibitors." In this way, affiliation with members away from the group reduces renewal. This concept may underlie

---

[5] 5 Only massive extinction trials have shown to be effective in a solitary exposure setting.

"sponsoring" in Alcoholics Anonymous in which a more seasoned group member is available to a new member for support on an individual basis. That is, the experienced member becomes a conditioned inhibitor by being in the group in which the less experienced member participates. In short, inhibitory conditioning can lead to increased generalization of the extinction phenomenon because nonthreatening cues counter previously threatening ones. In fact, the use of a conditioned inhibitor in extinction training has been shown to better immunize subjects against renewal than traditional extinction procedures without explicit inhibitor cues (Rauhut, Thomas, & Ayres, 2001).

Interestingly, conditioned inhibition is often used to explain why numerous extinction trials seem to lessen renewal (Denniston, Chang, & Miller, 2003). Massive extinction or exposure presentations may reduce the likelihood of renewal because they broaden the inhibitory generalization gradient. Thus, the patient that has undergone extended exposure treatment may better be able to access the inhibitory associations outside a specific extinction therapy context.

On a somewhat distant but related note, conditioned inhibition also can play a role in extinguishing avoidance behavior. That is, although fear responding may be acquired as a consequence of learned associations, it is maintained through negative reinforcement. The person avoids the feared context, thereby reducing the anxiety associated with the situation and preventing any opportunity for extinction. The act of avoidance creates a distinctive feedback loop whereby proprioceptive, spatial, visual, auditory, and tactile cues are used to secure negative reinforcement through avoidance of the feared US (Dinsmoor, 2001). Such avoidance leads to continued hypervigilance and apprehension and ensures successive reexperiencing of symptoms (Jones & Barlow, 1990). Because avoidance produces a period of safety, response feedback stimuli (e.g., physiological cues) may acquire conditioned inhibitory properties and become signals for the absence of threat (Domjan, 2003). These cues can actually reinforce avoidance behavior. Indeed, research finds that "safety-signal" stimuli, when made explicit, facilitate avoidance learning (Candido, Maldonado, & Vila, 1991; McAllister & McAllister, 1991). To extrapolate to exposure therapy, safety cues might be advantageously used to retard avoidance. For example, we might determine that a veteran's wife, three best friends, pets, and sentimental objects are safety-signal analogues that can be inserted in the exposure trials to facilitate extinction.

# CONCLUSION

Exposure therapy, derived from the extinction paradigm, presents the original trauma (US) in modified forms through imagery and verbalization accompanied by CS (e.g., setting, noises, weather, other people, etc.), some of which were originally associated with the trauma. However, even after exposure treatment, CS, present during the trauma event, may retain their power to reawaken trauma reactions when encountered in nonexposure contexts. Many clinicians continue to think that the US–CS connections are eradicated or replaced via exposure or extinction. They are not. They are only inhibited. Hence, the risk of renewal remains high if exposure treatment regimens are not maximized.

Contemporary learning theory suggests several methods for reducing the likelihood of renewal and optimizing exposure treatment, such as massive extinction trials. The use of numerous exposure trials, however, is contrary to the policy zeitgeist of the times, which entails brief therapy and managed care. Nevertheless, providing effective treatment at the outset of therapy may prevent relapse and thereby reduce the expense of treatment in the long run by preventing recurrent engagements.

The use of conditioned inhibition is another means by which to improve the effectiveness of exposure treatments. Cues present in exposure (e.g., music, smells, or even other people in the case of group exposures) can be invoked on subsequent occasions and in other contexts to maximize the generalization of extinction. Also, long-standing "safe" objects can be inserted in the exposure trials to more clearly signal the absence of danger. Family members, friends, pets, or a favorite song present during exposure can come to serve as a conditioned inhibitor of fear.

Finally, findings from behavioral studies suggest that nonreinforcement in the most surprising context possible, under conditions that closely approximate the original trauma, will make renewal less likely. Thus, the clinician should determine where the patient's reactions occur most frequently and intensely and then create the exposure context to contain relevant features. Furthermore, we think that a structured patient inquiry designed to establish trauma details will be fruitfully augmented by free association. Free association increases the likelihood that the web of associated memories linked to the trauma in the patient's experience will be more fully rendered. Admittedly, such a procedure needs refinement to discern when this "digging for details" has become asymptotic, else we run the risk of a never-ending hunt. However, the benefits would seem to outweigh the costs. In addition to elucidating the web of associations linked with the trauma responding, such an approach might also revive ideas that have come to b e attached to the trauma event. For example, the victim may make an attribution of self-blame regarding the event of the trauma or its aftermath. The attributions then lead us into the realm of cognitions, conceptual processing, and the meaning of trauma, a topic deserving separate discussion.

# REFERENCES

Bornstein, R. F. (1993). Implicit perception, implicit memory, and the recovery of unconscious material in psychotherapy. Journal of Nervous and Mental Disease, 181(6), 337–344.

Bouton, M. E. (1993). Context, time, and memory retrieval in the interference paradigms of Pavlovian learning. Psychological Bulletin, 114, 80–99.

Bouton, M. E. (1994). Conditioning, remembering, and forgetting. Journal of Experimental Psychology: Animal Behavior Processes, 20, 219–231.

Bouton, M. E., & Nelson, J. B. (1998). The role of context in classical conditioning: Some implications for cognitive behavior therapy. In W. O'Donohue (Ed.), Learning and behavior therapy (pp. 59–84). Boston: Allyn & Bacon.

Breslau, N. (1998). Epidemiology of trauma and posttraumatic stress disorder. In R. Yehuda (Ed.), Psychological trauma (pp. 1–29). Washington, DC: American Psychiatric Association.

Brewin, C. R., Dalgleish, T., & Joseph, S. (1996). A dual representation theory of posttraumatic stress disorder. Psychological Review, 103, 670–686.

Brewin, C. R., & Holmes, E. A. (2003). Psychological theories of posttraumatic stress disorder. Clinical Psychology Review, 23, 339–376.

Brooks, D. C., Palmatier, M. I., Garcia, E. O., & Johnson, J. L. (1999). An extinction cue reduces spontaneous recovery of conditioned taste aversion. Animal Learning and Behavior, 27, 77–88.

Candido, A., Maldonado, A., & Vila, J. (1991). Effects of duration of feedback on signaled avoidance. Animal Learning and Behavior, 19, 81–87.

Denniston, J. C., Chang, R. C., & Miller, R. R. (2003). Massive extinction treatment attenuates the renewal effect. Learning and Motivation, 34, 68–86.

Dinsmoor, J. A. (2001). Still no evidence for temporarily extended shock-frequency reduction as a reinforcer. Journal of the Experimental Analysis of Behavior, 75, 367–378.

Dollard, J., & Miller, N. E. (1950). Personality and psychotherapy. New York: McGraw-Hill, 1950.

Domjan, M. (2003). The principles of learning. Belmont, CA: Wadsworth/Thomas Learning.

Ehlers, A., & Clark, D. M. (2000). A cognitive model of posttraumatic stress disorder. Behavior Research and Theory, 38, 319–345.

Figley, C. R. (2002). Brief treatments for the traumatized: A project of the Green Cross Foundation: Vol. 39. Contributions in psychology. Westport, CT: Greenwood Press.

Foa, E. B., & Rothbaum, B. O. (2001). Treating the trauma of rape: Cognitive behavior therapy for PTSD. New York: Guilford Press.

Freud, S. (1953). The complete psychological works of Sigmund Freud (Vol. 3). London:Hogarth Press.

Halligan, S. L., Clark, D. M., & Ehlers, A. (2002). Cognitive processing, memory, and the 427 Exposure Therapy Renewed

development of PTSD symptoms: Two experimental analogue studies. Journal of Behavior Therapy and Experimental Psychiatry, 33, 73–89.

Halligan, S. L., Michael, T., Clark, D. M., & Ehlers, A. (2003). Posttraumatic stress disorder following assault: The role of cognitive processing, trauma memory, and appraisals.

Journal of Consulting and Clinical Psychology, 71(3), 419–431.

Jones, J. C., & Barlow, D. H. (1990). The etiology of posttraumatic stress disorder. Clinical Psychology Review, 10, 299–328.

Loftus, E. F. (1993). The reality of repressed memories. American Psychologist, 48, 518–537.

McAllister, D. E., & McAllister, W. R. (1991). Fear theory and aversively motivated behavior: Some controversial issues. In M. R. Denny (Ed.), Fear avoidance and phobias (pp. 135–163). Hillsdale, NJ: Erlbaum.

Murray, J., Ehlers, A., & Mayou, R. A. (2002). Dissociation and post-traumatic stress disorder: Two prospective studies of road traffic accident survivors. British Journal of

Psychiatry, 180, 363–368.

Paunovic, N. (1997). Exposure therapy for post-traumatic stress disorder: Its relative efficacy, limitations, and optimal application. Scandinavian Journal of Behavior Therapy, 26(2), 54–69.

Rauhut, A. S., Thomas, B. L., & Ayres, J. B. (2001). Treatments that weaken Pavlovian conditioned fear and thwart its renewal in rats: Implications for treating human phobias.

Journal of Experimental Psychology: Animal Behavior Processes, 27, 99–114.

Rescorla, R. A., & Wagner, A. R. (1972). A theory of Pavlovian conditioning: Variations in the effectiveness of reinforcement and nonreinforcement. In A. H. Black & W. F.

Prokasy (Eds.), Classical conditioning II: Current research and theory (pp. 64–99). New York: Appleton-Century-Crofts.

Rothbaum, B. O., & Schwartz, A. C. (2002). Exposure therapy for posttraumatic stress disorder. American Journal of Psychotherapy, 56(1), 59–75.

Thomas, B. L., Larsen, N., & Ayres, J. J. B. (2003). Role of context similarity in ABA, ABC, and AAB renewal paradigms: Implications for theories of renewal and for treating human phobias. Learning and Motivation, 34, 410–436.

Wilson, A., & Smith, F. J. (1968). Counterconditioning therapy using free association: A pilot study. Journal of Abnormal Psychology, 73(5), 474–478.

Wolberg, L. R. (1988). The technique of psychotherapy. Philadelphia: Gruen & Stratton. 428 Massad and Hulsey

# 11 Resolving Distress: Exposing A Medical Myth

## John Durkin

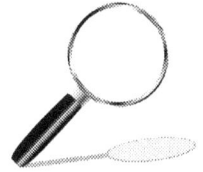

John Durkin is a psychologist specializing in stress-resolution and psychological growth. He is an accredited trainer in critical incident stress management and working toward his PhD in the School of Sociology & Social Policy at the University of Nottingham, UK. All correspondence to John Durkin via john@firestress.co.uk

## Abstract

The medical model, as it applies to psychological trauma, follows a similar model to addressing physical trauma in that it requires a set of symptoms to generate a diagnosis that proposes a specific course of treatment. The argument that the medical model may not be the most appropriate means to achieve the resolution of psychological trauma was made by the humanistic psychology movement. More recently, positive psychology has recognized the contribution of humanistic psychology in proposing a viewpoint that acknowledges a greater range of human experience than is possible through a focus on exclusively negative symptoms. If the medical model of psychological distress has ignored the positive aftermath of surviving adversity, then it may give an inadequate account of psychological trauma and so provide an incomplete model of resolution. In recognition of the positive as well as the negative consequences of traumatic experience, a brief, practical and clinically relevant measure of well-being will be introduced.

Positive psychological changes in the aftermath of distressing and difficult experiences have been recognized and discussed in many fields of human endeavour including literature, philosophy and religion (Tedeschi, Park & Calhoun, 1995). Empirical studies have been undertaken that have also demonstrated enhanced psychological health amongst those suffering a range of serious acute and chronic medical challenges including cancer, heart attack and addiction. One term that has been given to this adaptation to a range of threatening events is *adversarial growth* (Joseph & Linley, 2004). Clinicians have been urged to take account of the possibility of positive change in the aftermath of traumatic experience and were reminded that post-traumatic stress interventions rarely acknowledge adversarial growth even though it has been shown to be related to lower distress (Joseph & Linley, 2004).

# Positive Psychology and Growth through Adversity

Positive psychology is a movement incorporating the perspective of humanistic psychology as part of its foundation (Seligman, Steen, Park and Peterson, 2005) and resonant with the movement led by Rogers and Maslow in the 1950s and 1960s (Joseph & Linley, 2006). The humanistic movement, in its person-centered view, acknowledges the range of human experience in the encounter with psychological distress and relies on the assumption of an innate tendency towards growth to explain resolution from distress. This compares with the medical model focus of categorizing distress by symptom clusters and offering treatment for negative symptoms where the patient's role in recovery may be overlooked. This bias towards the negative features of traumatic experience has drawn criticism from some positive psychologists who argue against the *medicalization* of such experience (e.g. Maddux, Snyder & Lopez, 2004). The medical model viewpoint however, is seemingly a very influential one given its appearance in some authoritative guidance on treatment for Post-traumatic Stress Disorder (PTSD) considered below.

# Treatment Guidelines for Post-traumatic Stress Disorder

In March 2005 the National Institute for Clinical Excellence (NICE) issued guidelines to the National Health Service in the United Kingdom (UK) on the treatment of PTSD. Treatment recommendations were restricted to Trauma-Focused Cognitive-Behavioral Therapy (TF-CBT), Eye-Movement Desensitization And Reprocessing (EMDR) and drug therapies where TF-CBT or EDMR proved unsuccessful. Early in the guidelines the authors offer the following advice:

Initial response to trauma

- For individuals who have experienced a traumatic event, the systematic provision to that individual alone of brief, single-session interventions (often referred to as debriefing) that focus on the traumatic incident, should not be routine practice when delivering services.

- Where symptoms are mild and have been present for less than 4 weeks after the trauma, watchful waiting, as a way of managing the difficulties presented by people with post-traumatic stress disorder (PTSD), should be considered. A follow-up contact should be arranged within 1 month (NICE, 2005, p. 123).

The first point warns against the use of an intervention called "debriefing" although no definition of debriefing was given in the guidelines. Reference was made however, to a Cochrane Review (Rose, Bisson, Churchill & Wessely, 2002). Rose et al. (2002), investigating psychological debriefing for preventing Post-traumatic Stress Disorder. The review reported two studies with negative outcomes; one study showed no benefit and the other suggested the prospect of harm. Both were carried out on hospital patients even though no precedent for debriefing hospital patients has been unearthed. Critical Incident Stress Debriefing (Mitchell, 1983) - a structured, group-based intervention initially developed for emergency personnel – was nevertheless cited, adapted and used in those studies. To those familiar with the *Mitchell-model* the irrelevance of studies reporting the effects of debriefing individual, hospitalized casualties idea will not be lost. Additionally a return to function is a stated aim of crisis-intervention techniques, which, if the focus of a psychological investigation is to be thoroughly assessed, should be measured. While a positive-model view might anticipate such progress, the medical model view may simply overlook restored function, especially when remnants of negative symptoms persist. In the absence of a meaningful measurement of recovery, debate is reduced to the conundrum of whether the glass is half-empty or half-full.

The second point recommends "watchful waiting" for up to four weeks after a traumatic incident for those who present with symptoms. Waiting one month for a follow-up - another unspecified procedure - was not explained but does coincide with the duration criterion between event and symptom manifestation that would justify a diagnosis of PTSD according to the DSM-IV (American Psychological Association, 1994). In practice it would appear that beyond the observation of emergent symptoms during the post-incident period, no intervention is recommended.

## Crisis Intervention

The practice of crisis-intervention has been described and reported since the First World War when the principles of *Immediacy, Proximity and Expectancy* were advanced to promote the idea of acting quickly to restore normality in soldiers following combat (Salmon, 1919, p. 993). These principles are the foundation of Critical Incident Stress Management (CISM) training programs which advocate peer-support as the psychosocial medium through which crisis-intervention be undertaken (Everly and Mitchell, 1999). CISM can be regarded as a person-centered approach as it presumes little expertise on the part of the interventionist for knowledge of the other's condition, but seeks to provide the safe environment necessary for the affected individual to express themselves frankly and authentically. Creating conditions for the successful resolution of psychological trauma has been proposed by Herman (1992). These conditions begin with the establishment of safety as the fundamental first step. Once established, safety can lead to the processes of remembrance and mourning followed by reconnection with those from whom the survivor has become estranged. This presents a schema for outlining how recovery is supported and encouraged. Recovery may be enhanced if the cognitive and emotional elements of the experience can be appreciated in a supportive environment to generate additional meaning. It is such progress that can lead to new understanding and ultimately, psychological growth.

## Traumatic Incident Reduction

Traumatic Incident Reduction (TIR; Gerbode, 1995) is a structured, parsimonious, person-centered approach for resolving stress in emotionally-distressed individuals. Whereas the medicalization of traumatic stress has led to the perception that helping people overcome the effects of adverse experiences requires highly-trained and expert intervention, proponents of the TIR approach argue that distress following adverse experiences is indicative of normal processes of recovery that require little more than an interested listener and a commitment to a strictly person-centered procedure (Gerbode, 1995).

In the NICE guidelines discussed above, the medical view is apparent in that access to treatment is made following diagnosis. It was noted however, that problematic symptoms have to emerge in order to justify a diagnosis as only "watchful waiting" was advised for four weeks post-event. Depending on the availability of treatment resources an indefinite wait could ensue. Not only could this waiting period allow a worsening of distress, but it would deny other forms of intervention that might bring some benefit. Offering a treatment regimen based entirely on the emergence of negative consequences is likely to paint an incomplete picture of the experience of the individual. In the view of those who employ person-centered practices such as crisis-intervention and TIR, to present a diagnosis is to medicalize a normal recovery process. It is foreseeable that to diagnose and so describe the early stages of recovery as a mental illness, with the associated stigma, might undermine the efforts of some sufferers to address their current problems. Alternatively, seeing distress on a continuum of well-being, rather than as the presence or absence of negative symptoms, would at least acknowledge the presence of positive elements in the recovery process that are overlooked in a medical search for pathology.

## Assessing Psychological Well-being

Acknowledgement of a continuum of functioning with negative aspects at one end and positive aspects at the other would enable, with appropriate measurement, the recognition of movement along that continuum as a means to monitoring recovery. Such a measurement tool, has been described in the development of the Short Depression Happiness Scale (SDHS: Joseph, Linley, Harwood, Lewis & McCollam, 2004). The SDHS was developed from items selected from the original Depression Happiness Scale (Joseph & Lewis, 1998), a 25-item scale that offered a continuous measure of depression and happiness with both variables lying along a continuum. The six items of the SDHS were scored and computed against scores on the Beck Depression Inventory (BDI: Beck & Steer, 1987) ($r = -.63, p < .0001$) and the Oxford Happiness Inventory (OHI: Argyle, Martin, & Crossland, 1989) ($r = .69, p < .001$) demonstrating the convergent validity of the SDHS as a measurement tool for depression and happiness. It was reported that of 21 participants who scored 10 or higher on the BDI ($M = 15.76, SD = 4.83$) their median score on the SDHS were about 9 ($M = 9.43, SD = 2.87$) suggesting that a score of 10 on the SDHS would present a cut-off for mild, but clinically relevant depression. As the SDHS is negatively correlated with the BDI, lower scores would indicate increasing depressive symptoms.

The SDHS correlates well with both the BDI and the OHI and the scale uses six statements with a 0-3 response scale for each statement giving a 0-18 scoring range (statements 1, 3 & 6 score 3, 2, 1 & 0 while statements 2, 4 & 5 are reversed). Low scores on the SDHS correlate with depressive symptoms while higher scores represent increasing happiness. This brief measure allows for the rapid measurement of overall psychological well-being. Repeated measurements would identify movement along the continuum with increasing scores to indicate recovery and growth, or with decreasing scores to identify ongoing difficulties.

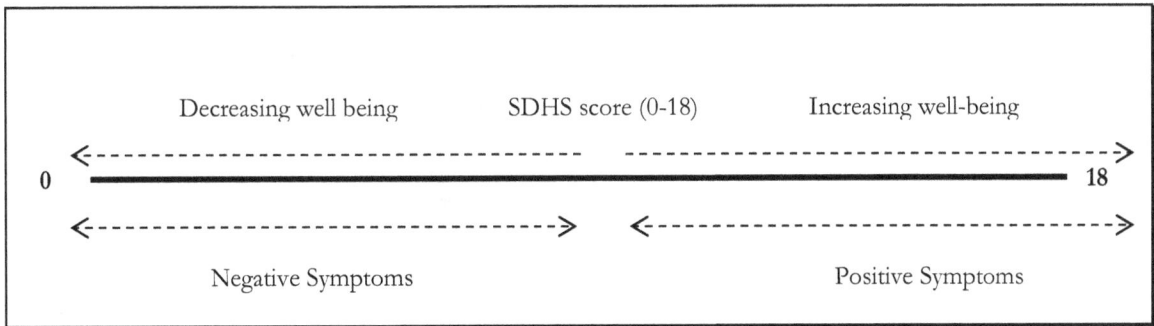

**Fig.1: Continuum of functioning measured by Short Depression Happiness Scale**

## Conclusion

Alternative paradigms to the medical model of traumatic experience can benefit from the employment of the SDHS as the post-traumatic aftermath unfolds. Not only is there measurement of a greater range of emotional expression than clinical measures allow but the defining assumption of the humanistic movement that individuals are intrinsically motivated towards growth and fulfillment can find some expression in such an assessment tool. A number of psychotherapeutic or interventionist approaches could see their effects measured quickly and effectively using the SDHS and be used to initiate empirical evidence of benefit that are currently lacking.

Practitioners of TIR have been invited to employ the SDHS formally in order to give weight to their success with their person-centered methods and to generate empirical evidence of change following sessions. While evaluations of success within the medical model are bound by the limitations of measuring the reduction of negative symptoms, they invariably overlook features of positive adaptation and growth in those challenged by the setback of an adverse life-event. Clinical guidance that relies on the detection of pathological symptoms as the primary focus for resolving traumatic stress, may present an inadequate understanding of how people respond to their experience of traumatic episodes. The SDHS can be applied in numerous post-trauma settings to measure both the reduction in negative symptoms and the positive improvements in well-being.

## The Short Depression-Happiness Scale (SDHS: Joseph, Linley, Harwood, Lewis & McCollam, 2004)

A number of statements that people have made to describe how they feel are given below. Please read each one and tick the box which best describes how frequently you feel that way in the **past seven days, including today**. Some statements describe positive feelings and some negative feelings. You may have experienced both positive and negative feelings at different times during the past seven days.

|  | Never | Rarely | Some-times | Often |
|---|---|---|---|---|
| (1)  I felt dissatisfied with my life |  |  |  |  |
| (2)  I felt happy |  |  |  |  |
| (3)  I felt cheerless |  |  |  |  |
| (4)  I felt pleased with the way I am |  |  |  |  |
| (5)  I felt that life was enjoyable |  |  |  |  |
| (6)  I felt that life was meaningless |  |  |  |  |

# References

American Psychiatric Association (1994). *Diagnostic and statistical manual of mental disorders.* (4th ed.). Washington, DC: Author.

Argyle, M., Martin, M., & Crossland, J. (1989). Happiness as a function of personality and social encounters. In J. P. Forgas & J. M. Innes (Eds). *Recent advances in social psychology: An inter-national perspective.* North Holland: Elsevier.

Beck, A.T. & Steer, R.A. (1987). *Beck Depression Inventory Manual.* San Antonio, TX: The Psychological Corporation.

Everly, G.S. & Mitchell, J.T. (1999). *Critical Incident Stress Management: A New Era and Standard of Care in Crisis Intervention.* (2nd ed.). Ellicott City, MD: Chevron Publishing Corporation.

Gerbode, F.A. (1995). *Beyond Psychology: An Introduction to Metapsychology.* (3rd Ed.). Menlo Park, CA: IRM Press.

Herman, J.L. (1992). *Trauma and Recovery.* New York: Basic Books

Joseph, S., & Lewis, C. A. (1998). The Depression-Happiness Scale: Reliability and validity of a bipolar self-report scale. *Journal of Clinical Psychology, 54,* 537-544.

Joseph, S., Linley, P. A., Harwood, J., Lewis, C. A., & McCollam, P. (2004). Rapid assessment of well-being: The Short Depression-Happiness Scale (SDHS). *Psychology and Psychotherapy: Theory, Research and Practice, 77,* 463-478.

Joseph, S., & Linley, P. A. (2006). Positive psychology versus the medical model. *American Psychologist, 61,* 332-333.

Joseph, S., & Worsley, R. (2005). *Person-centered psychopathology: A positive psychology of mental health.* Ross-on-Wye: PCCS books.

Maddux, J.E., Snyder, C.R. & Lopez S.J. (2004). Toward a positive clinical psychology: Deconstructing the illness ideology and constructing an ideology of human strengths and potential. In P.A. Lindley & S. Joseph (Eds). *Positive Psychology in Practice.* Hoboken, NJ: John Wiley.

Mitchell, J.T. (1983). When disaster strikes…the critical incident stress debriefing process. *Journal of Emergency Medical Services, 8,* 36–39

National Institute for Clinical Excellence (2005). *Post-traumatic Stress Disorder: The management of PTSD in adults and children in primary and secondary care.* National Clinical Practice Guideline Number 26. London: Gaskell & British Psychological Society.

Rose, S., Bisson, J., Churchill, R. &, Wessely, S. (2002). Psychological debriefing for preventing post traumatic stress disorder (PTSD). *Cochrane Database of Systematic Reviews: Reviews 2002 Issue 2* Chichester, UK: John Wiley & Sons, Ltd.

Salmon, T.S. (1919). War neuroses and their lesson. *New York Medical Journal, 109,* 993-994.

Seligman, M.E.P., Steen, T.A., Park, N. & Peterson, C. (2005). Positive psychology progress: Empirical validation of interventions. *American Psychologist, 60,* 410-421.

Tedeschi RG, Calhoun LG (1995). *Trauma & Transformation: Growing in the Aftermath of Suffering.* Thousand Oaks, CA: Sage Publications.

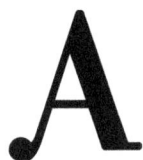

# A Bibliography and Resources

## Dissertations on or Involving TIR

Research papers available from Dissertation Express are indicated with Order Numbers in the list below.

- Bisbey, L., (January, 1995). "No Longer a Victim: a Treatment Outcome Study of Crime Victims with Post-Traumatic Stress Disorder." (Doctoral Dissertation, California School of Professional Psychology, San Diego, CA.)
[Ed. Note: Her dissertation compared TIR and Imaginal Flooding with a control group with 57 subjects]
Specify Order Number 9522269
- Coughlin, W., (May, 1995). "Traumatic Incident Reduction: Efficacy in Reducing Anxiety Symptomatology." (Doctoral Dissertation, Union Institute, Cincinnati, OH.) Specify Order Number 9537919
- Odio, Francine (2003) "Traumatic Incident Reduction (TIR) Program for Children." (Doctoral Dissertation, Carlos Albizu University.)
Publication Number AAT 3100829 from Digital Dissertations
- Valentine, Pamela V. (1997) "Traumatic Incident Reduction: Brief Treatment of Trauma-Related Symptoms in Incarcerated Females." (Doctoral Dissertation, Florida State University. Advisor: Smith, Thomas E.)
Specify Order Number 9725020

Students, faculty, staff and researchers can order their own unbound copies of dissertations and theses with express delivery to their home, school or office. Select from over one million titles available from UMI by visiting http://wwwlib.umi.com/dxweb/

# Metapsychology/TIR–Related Literature

**In order of publication date:**

Gerbode, F.A. (1989). *Beyond Psychology: an Introduction to Metapsychology*, 3rd Ed. (1995) Menlo Park, CA: IRM Press

Moore, R.H. (1992). "Cognitive-Emotive Treatment of the Post-Traumatic Stress Disorder". In W. Dryden and L. Hill (Eds.) *Innovations in Rational-Emotive Therapy*. Newbury Park, CA: Sage Publications

Moore, R.H. (1993). "Innovative Techniques for Practitioners". *The RET Resource Book for Practitioners*. New York, NY: Institute for Rational-Emotive Therapy.

Gerbode, F.A. & Moore, R.H. (1994). "Beliefs and Intentions in RET." *Journal of Rational-Emotive & Cognitive-Behavior Therapy*, Vol. 12, No. 1., Albert Ellis Institute

French, Gerald D., MA, CTS and Harris, Chrys, Ph.D., CTS (1998), *Traumatic Incident Reduction (TIR)*. CRC Press

Bisbey, L., MA, CTS and Bisbey, S. (1999) *Brief Therapy for Post-Traumatic Stress Disorder: Traumatic Incident Reduction and Related Technique*. John Wiley & Sons.

Descilo, Teresa (1999) "Relieving the Traumatic Aspects of Death with Traumatic Incident Reduction and EMDR". In: pp. 153-182; Figley, Charles R [ed.]; *Traumatology of Grieving: Conceptual, Theoretical, and Treatment Foundations*; Philadelphia: Brunner/Mazel,

Gerbode, F.A. (2005). "Traumatic Incident Reduction" in Garrick and Williams [ed.] *Trauma Treatment Techniques: Innovative Trends*. New York, NY: Haworth Press.

Volkman, Marian (2005) *Life Skills: Improve the Quality of Your Life with Metapsychology*. Ann Arbor, MI. Loving Healing Press.

Volkman, Victor (2005) *Beyond Trauma: Conversations on Traumatic Incident Reduction, 2nd Ed.* Ann Arbor, MI. Loving Healing Press.

Volkman, Victor (2005) *Traumatic Incident Reduction: Research and Results*. Ann Arbor, MI. Loving Healing Press.

Volkman, Victor (2006) *Traumatic Incident Reduction and Critical Incident Stress Management: A Synergistic Approach*. Ann Arbor, MI. Loving Healing Press

Volkman, Marian (2007) *Children and Traumatic Incident Reduction: Creative and Cognitive Approaches*. Ann Arbor, MI. Loving Healing Press.

Volkman, Victor (2008) *Traumatic Incident Reduction: Research and Results, 2nd Ed.* .Ann Arbor, MI. Loving Healing Press.

French, Gerald D., MA, CTS and Harris, Chrys, Ph.D., CTS (2008), *Traumatic Incident Reduction (TIR), 2nd Ed.* Ann Arbor, MI. Loving Healing Press

# Selected Mentions of TIR in Trauma Literature

*Coping with Post-Traumatic Stress Disorder: A Guide for Families*, by Cheryl A. Roberts, McFarland & Company, 2003 ISBN 0786417366 , pp. 96-97 (Chapter 7 discusses EMDR and TIR)

*Brief Treatments for the Traumatized: A Project of the Green Cross Foundation* , edited by Charles R Figley, 2002, CRC Press ISBN: 031332137X, pp. 252-265 (Chapter 12 by Pamela Vest Valentine, Ph.D. on TIR)

*Got Parts? An Insider's Guide to Managing Life Successfully with Dissociative Identity Disorder*, by A.T.W, 2005 ISBN 1932690034, Loving Healing Press. p. 170. mentions TIR as a possible handling for DID clients who are ready for it.

*Energy Psychology*, by Fred P. Gallo, ISBN 574441841, CRC Press. pp. 18-23 on TIR and three other techniques studies in Figley's "Active Ingredient" project. 1998

*Not Trauma Alone: Therapy for Child Abuse Survivors in Family and Social Context*, Steven L. Gold, pp. 220-227 recommends TIR for use with survivors of PCA (Prolonged Child Abuse). ISBN: 1583910271, Brunner-Routledge. 2000

"Creating a Comprehensive Trauma Center : Choices and Challenges" by Mary Beth Williams, Lasse A. Nurmi, ISBN 030646327X, .Plenum Press. p. 38 indicates that "TIR may be effective for uncomplicated PTSD." 2001.

*Trauma: A Practitioners Guide to Counselling*, by Thom Spiers, ISBN: 0415186943. Brunner-Routledge. 2002. p. 119 says that "Clients who have a tendency to cut off from their feelings when talking about the incident may benefit from TIR." There are a few other mentions throughout the book.

*Bullying and Emotional Abuse in the Workplace: International Perspectives in Research and Practice* by Cary Cooper, p.276 article by Noreen Tehrani "illustrates how TIR help a manager deal with the painful memory of a difficult team meeting." with actual session dialog. ISBN 0415253594, CRC Press, 2002.

*Crisis Intervention Handbook: Assessment, Treatment, and Research* Ed by Albert R. Roberts, ISBN: 019513365X, Oxford University Press, 2000. has a chapter by Pamela Vest Valentine, Ph.D. on Adult Survivors of Incest: p. 265 states that "Both TIR and group treatment have been tested and found effective in assisting clients in answering old questions and generating new options".

*Peak States of Consciousness: Theory and Applications, Volume 1: Breakthrough Techniques for Exceptional Quality of Life* by McFetridge, Aldana, Hardt and Slavinski (2004)

"Although as laymen we tend to think of trauma as extending over time, in reality trauma is composed of discrete moments in time. These moments often form a chain of traumatic moments linked by their sensation content. Several therapies take advantage of this fact in healing, such as Body-Centered Therapy by Gay Hendricks, Traumatic Incident Reduction by Frank Gerbode, and my own Whole-Hearted Healing." ( p.65 )

Oz, S., Eitan, M., & Motzkin, K. (2005). The wall of fear: The bridge between the traumatic event and trauma resolution therapy for childhood sexual abuse survivors. *Journal of Child Sexual Abuse*. 14:3,

> *Simple and Complex Post-Traumatic Stress Disorder: Strategies for Comprehensive Treatment in Clinical Practice* by Mary Beth Williams SBN: 0789002981, Haworth Press. 2002. Chapter 12. by Chrys J. Harris, M.D. p. 270 "Using TIR as the treatment of choice for the family members when there is vicarious, chiasmal, or intra-family trauma should allow the family therapist to treat the individual family members in a relatively brief time."

> *Counselling Individuals: A Rational Emotive Behavioural Handbook*, 4th Ed. 2005 by Windy Dryden, Michael Neenan. Mentions that TIR is effective for PTSD symptoms.

> *Depth Oriented Brief Therapy (DOBT) : How to Be Brief When You Were Trained to Be Deep and Vice Versa* (Jossey Bass Social and Behavioral Science Series) ISBN: 0787901520, pub date 1995 by Bruce Ecker on page 217:

"Traumatic Incident Reduction (TIR) is a technique developed by psychotherapists Frank Gerbode and Gerald French for fundamentally resolving (rather than merely managing or controlling) post-traumatic stress symptomatology. It is a process for rapidly accessing and dispelling the unconscious traumatic constructions of reality set up by the client during a traumatic event."

"In DOBT terms, the TIR technique efficiently carries out radical inquiry and position work in relation to a particular type of pro-symptom position, one in which the (ongoing) emotional reality was formed by a traumatic incident. This repetitive, detailed, subjective review instigates a thorough emotional processing of this memory, progressively filling in lost details and unfolding the crucial moments of meaning-formation that occurred during the incident. This brings about a spontaneous emergence into awareness of the symptom-generating meanings, construals, intentions, and protective actions that were unconsciously formed. Thus, the TIR process fits very well within the DOBT framework of psychotherapy"

# Selected Journal Articles about TIR

Commons, Michael L. "The Power Therapies: a Proposed Mechanism for their Action and Suggestions for Future Empirical Validation" .*Traumatology*, 6(2): pp. 119-138, August 2000, ISSN: 1534-7656

Dietrich, Anne M; Baranowsky, Anna B; Devich-Navarro, Mona; Gentry, J Eric; Harris, Chrys Jay; Figley, Charles R "A review of alternative approaches to the treatment of post traumatic sequelae." *Traumatology*, 6(4): pp. 251-271, December 2000, ISSN: 1534-7656

Figley, Charles R; Carbonnell, Joyce L; Boscarino, Joseph A; Chang, Jeani. "A Clinical Demonstration Model for Assessing the Effectiveness of Therapeutic Interventions: an Expanded Clinical Trials Methodology." *International Journal of Emergency Mental Health*, 1(3): pp. 155-164, Summer 1999

Gallo, Fred P. "Reflections on active ingredients in efficient treatments of PTSD, part 2." *Traumatology*, 2(2): pp. [Article 2], 1996 ISSN: 1534-7656

Mitchels, B. (2003). "Healing the wounds of war and more: an integrative approach to peace--the work of Adam Curle and others with Mir I. Dobro in Upanja, Croatia". *British Journal of Guidance and Counselling*, 31(4), 403-416.

Valentine, P. and Smith, Thomas E. "Evaluating Traumatic Incident Reduction Therapy with Female Inmates: a Randomized Controlled Clinical Trial." *Research on Social Work Practice*, v. 11, no. 1, pp. 40-52, January 2001, ISSN: 1049-7315

Valentine, P. "Traumatic Incident Reduction I: Traumatized Women Inmates: Particulars of Practice and Research", *Journal of Offender Rehabilitation* Vol. 31(3-4): 1-15, 2000

Valentine, P. and Smith, Thomas E. "A Qualitative Study of Client Perceptions of Traumatic Incident Reduction (TIR): a Brief Trauma Treatment." *Crisis Intervention and Time-Limited Treatment*, v. 4, no. 1, pp. 1-12, 1998, ISSN: 1064-5136

Valentine, P. "Traumatic Incident Reduction: A Review of a New Intervention." *Journal of Family Psychotherapy*, 6, (2), 79-85, 1995.

Wylie, M. S. "Researching PTSD: Going for the Cure." *Family Therapy Networker*, 20(4), pp. 20-37, July/Aug. 1996.

# AMI/TIRA Newsletter Compendium

Although not a peer-reviewed research journal, the *AMI/TIRA Newsletter* (ISSN 1555-0818) frequently contains insightful interviews of TIR practitioners working in the field as well as background theory pieces on principles of Metapsychology. Requests for electronic or paper reprints may be directed to ami@TIR.org. The AMI/TIRA Newsletter (2004-present) subsumes the role of its predecessors: TIRA News and Views Newsletter (1998-2003) and the Newsletter of the Institute for Research in Metapsychology (1989-97). Reprints of the latter can be found in *Beyond Trauma: Conversations on TIR, 2nd Ed.* (2005). The following compendium covers *AMI/TIRA Newsletter* up to the point of publication of this volume (April 2005).

Volkman, V. (2004). Dr. Anna B. Baranowsky and the traumatology institute of canada. *AMI/TIRA Newsletter, 1*(1), 4-5.

Volkman, M. (2004). TIR certification streamlining in 2004. *AMI/TIRA Newsletter, 1*(1), 6.

Volkman, M. (2004). Two simple remedies for children. *AMI/TIRA Newsletter, 1*(2), 5-6.

Volkman, V. (2004). Counseling inmates: a conversation with John Nielsen. *AMI/TIRA Newsletter, 1*(2), 7-10.

Volkman, V. (2004). TIR and dissociative identity disorder: a conversation with Aerial Long, cmf, ct. *AMI/TIRA Newsletter, 1*(3), 2-4, 8.

Volkman, M. (2004). Deepening client engagement. *AMI/TIRA Newsletter, 1*(3), 6-7.

Volkman, V. (2004). TIR in a mental health clinic setting: a conversation with Patricia Furze, msw, rsw. *AMI/TIRA Newsletter, 1*(4), 3-4, 9-12.

Peacock, S. (2004). Relaxation/visualization exercise. *AMI/TIRA Newsletter, 1*(4), 6-7.

Volkman, M. (2005). Resilience, defenses, and case progress. *AMI/TIRA Newsletter, 2*(1), 3.

Volkman, V. (2005). TIR in the workplace: a conversation with Wendy Kruger. *AMI/TIRA Newsletter, 2*(1), 6-10.

Gerbode, F. A. (2005). Reality and the person-centered approach. *AMI/TIRA Newsletter, 2*(2), 4-7, 11-13.

Volkman, V. (2005). Miami TIR experts train tsunami relief workers. *AMI/TIRA Newsletter, 2*(2), 8-10.

Volkman, V. (2005). TIR in a Victim Services Agency: A Conversation with Joanna Woodd, Victim Services Lambeth. *AMI/TIRA Newsletter, 2*(3), 4-6.

Volkman, V. (2005) TIR & Art Therapy: A Conversation with Anna Foley. *AMI/TIRA Newsletter, 2*(4), 7-12.

Velazquez-Garcia, C. (2005). Critical Incident Stress Debriefing and TIR Training: Strange Bedfellows or Soulmates? *AMI/TIRA Newsletter*, *2*(4), 17-20.

Gerbode, F.A. (2006). A Metapsychological View of ADHD and OCD. *AMI/TIRA Newsletter*, *3*(1), 4-5, 9-12.

Durkin, J. (2006). Traumatic Incident Reduction: From Observation to Evidence. *AMI/TIRA Newsletter*, *3*(1), 7-8.

Volkman, M. (2006). Presence and Intention. *AMI/TIRA Newsletter*, *3*(1), 13-14.

Canant, D. (2006). Looking for Common Ground. *AMI/TIRA Newsletter*, *3*(2), 3-6, 17-18.

Volkman, M. (2006). A Theory of Destructive Behavior. *AMI/TIRA Newsletter*, *3*(2), 7-10.

Gerbode, F. (2006). An Introduction to the Metapsychology Curriculum. *AMI/TIRA Newsletter*, *3*(2), 13-16.

Day, N. (2006). Critical Incident Stress Management and TIR. *AMI/TIRA Newsletter*, *3*(3), 5-11.

Volkman, M. (2006). The Value of Material Objects for Clients in Session. *AMI/TIRA Newsletter*, *3*(3), 14-15.

# Web Resources

The primary location of all TIR literature on the Internet continues to be the www.TIR.org website. Below are listed some key pages containing material currently out-of-print in any other milieu:

## Essays on TIR and Metapsychology

Includes a dozen essays by Frank A. Gerbode, M.D., the primary developer of Metapsychology. Also included is both introductory material and a case study by Robert H. Moore, Ph.D.

See http://www.tir.org/metapsy/essay_menu.htm

## Case Studies and TIR

Read about how practitioners are using TIR and related methods to help clients resolve their issues. Highlights specific groups including Vietnam veterans, crime victims and inmates, accident victims, terrorism survivors, dissociative identity disorder survivors, and prenatal/perinatal trauma.

See http://www.tir.org/metapsy/case_menu.htm

## Journal of Metapsychology: Selected Reprints (1986–1997)

Many of the early JOM articles here both influenced and were integrated into Dr. Gerbode's book *Beyond Psychology: An Introduction to Metapsychology, 3rd, Ed.* (1995). An additional project is underway to revise and reprint as many of the 112 articles as possible. Contact info@tir.org for latest details.

See http://www.tir.org/metapsy/jom/000_intro.html for online JOM articles.

# The TIR and Metapsychology Lecture Series

The TIR and Metapsychology Lecture Series gathers together for the first time all of the seminal lectures of Frank A. Gerbode, M.D., the developer of TIR and theorist of Metapsychology. Dr. Gerbode's self-effacing and conversational style along with his solid expertise in Traumatology have made him a favorite among conference attendees. The following volumes are recommended listening from Loving Healing Press (www.LovingHealing.com):

| | TIR and Metapsychology Lecture Series<br>Vol. M1: Gerbode on TIR and Metapsychology | | |
|---|---|---|---|
| Track | Title/Notes | Year | Time |
| 1 | An Anamnestic Approach to Trauma (1 of 2)<br>with Gerald French<br>and Charles Figley, Ph.D | 1994 | 60 min |
| 2 | An Anamnestic Approach to Trauma (2 of 2)<br>with Gerald French<br>and Charles Figley, Ph.D | 1994 | 30 min |
| 3 | Seeing Beyond [interview]: (1 of 2)<br>with Robert Moore, Ph.D | 1992 | 60 min |
| 4 | Seeing Beyond [interview]: (2 of 2) | 1992 | 40 min |
| 5 | Empathy Workshop (1 of 2) | 1993 | 60 min |
| 6 | Empathy Workshop (2 of 2) | 1993 | 30 min |
| 7 | On the Nature of Hope | 1988 | 60 min |
| 8 | The Mind as Environment | 1993 | 53 min |
| 9 | Trauma and How to Resolve it (1 of 2)<br>with Robert Moore, Ph.D<br>and David B. Cheek, M.D. | 1991 | 43 min |
| 10 | Trauma and How to Resolve it (2 of 2)<br>with Robert Moore, Ph.D<br>and David B. Cheek, M.D. | 1991 | 41 min |
| 11 | The Purpose of Viewing | 1991 | 50 min |
| 12 | Applied Metapsychology: Therapy<br>or Personal Growth?** | 1995 | 24 min |
| 13 | Why Metapsychology? | 1989 | 60 min |

**As featured in the book *Beyond Trauma: Conversations on Traumatic Incident Reduction*

| TIR and Metapsychology Lecture Series<br>Vol. M5: Moore on TIR and Metapsychology | | | |
|:---:|:---|:---:|:---:|
| Track | Title/Notes | Year | Time |
| 1 | Introduction to TIR | | 71 min |
| 2 | Critical Issues in Trauma Resolution (1 of 4)<br>with Frank A. Gerbode, M.D. | | 79 min |
| 3 | Critical Issues in Trauma Resolution (2 of 4) | | 79 min |
| 4 | Critical Issues in Trauma Resolution (3 of 4) | | 45 min |
| 5 | Critical Issues in Trauma Resolution (4 of 4) | | 46 min |
| 6 | Trauma and How to Resolve it (1 of 2)<br>with Robert Moore, Ph.D<br>and David B. Cheek, M.D. | 1991 | 43 min |
| 7 | Trauma and How to Resolve it (2 of 2)<br>with Robert Moore, Ph.D<br>and David B. Cheek, M.D. | 1991 | 41 min |
| 8 | Group Discussion on Improving your Practice | | 71 min |
| 9 | Plenary address to IRM Conference | 1988 | 75 min |
| 10 | A Conversation with Robert Moore, Ph.D** | 2003 | 10 min |

**As featured in the book *Beyond Trauma: Conversations on Traumatic Incident Reduction*

# B Frequently Asked Questions (FAQs)

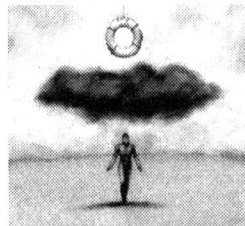

This section should answer some questions for professional practitioners (clinical psychologists, social workers, counselors, therapists, ministers, etc.) interested in using TIR & related techniques. Others should consider reading the **FAQ for Those Interested in Receiving TIR & Related Techniques** available on the website www.TIR.org.

## FAQ for Practitioners Interested in Using TIR & Related Techniques

### Contents:

1. What is TIR?
2. What is TIR Useful for?
3. How long has TIR been in use?
4. What is the anticipated outcome of TIR?
5. What are the contraindications and risks of TIR?
6. What are the historical antecedents of TIR?
7. How and why does TIR work?
8. How does TIR compare with other techniques for addressing traumatic stress?
9. How can I find out more about TIR?
10. How can one get trained in TIR?
11. What are the prerequisites for training?
12. How can I refer people to a TIR practitioner?

# 1. What is TIR?

TIR is a brief, one-on-one, non-hypnotic, person-centered, simple and highly structured method for permanently eliminating the negative effects of past traumas. It involves repeated viewing of a traumatic memory under conditions designed to enhance safety and minimize distractions. The client does the most important work in the session; the therapist or counselor offers no interpretations or negative or positive evaluations, but only gives appropriate instructions to the client to have him view a traumatic incident thoroughly from beginning to end. Hence, we use the term "viewer" to describe the client and "facilitator" to describe the person who is helping the client through the procedure by keeping the structure of the session intact and giving the viewer something definite to do at all times. The facilitator confines herself simply to giving a series of set instructions to the viewer; she offers no advice, interpretations, evaluations, or reassurances.

In what we call Basic TIR, which addresses known incidents, the viewer locates a specific trauma that he is interested in working on—one with a specific, finite duration. Then he treats the incident like a "videotape". First, he "rewinds" it to the beginning, then "plays" it through to the end—without talking about it while he is viewing it. *After* he has viewed it, the facilitator then asks him what happened, and he can then describe the event or his reactions to going through it.

After the viewer has completed one viewing (and one description), the facilitator has him "rewind the videotape" to the beginning and run through it again in the same fashion. The facilitator does not prescribe the degree of detail or content the viewer is to get on each run-through. The viewer will view as much as he is relatively comfortable viewing. After several run-throughs, most viewers will be able to contact the emotion and uncomfortable details in terms of the strengths of the emotion more thoroughly. Typically, the viewer will reach an emotional peak after a few run-throughs and then, on successive run-throughs, the amount of negative emotion will diminish, until the viewer reaches a point of having no negative emotion about the incident. Instead, he becomes rather thoughtful and contemplative, and usually comes up with one or more insights concerning the trauma, life, or himself. He displays positive emotion, often smiling or laughing, but at least manifesting calm and serenity. At this point, the viewer has reached an "end point" and the facilitator stops the TIR procedure.

In Thematic TIR, a specific feeling called a "theme" is used to discharge a sequence of related traumatic incidents.

A TIR session is not ended until the viewer reaches an end point and feels good. This may take anywhere from a few minutes to 3-4 hours. Average session time for a new viewer is about 90 minutes. Average total session hours to eliminate PTSD symptoms is 15 - 20 hours.

## 2. What is TIR useful for?

It is highly effective in eliminating the negative effects of past traumatic incidents. It is especially useful when:

a. A person has a specific trauma or set of traumas that she feels has adversely affected her, whether or not she has received a format diagnosis of "PTSD".

b. A person reacts inappropriately or overreacts in certain situations, and it is thought some past trauma might have something to do with it.

c. A person experiences unaccountable or inappropriate negative emotions, either chronically or in response to certain experiential triggers.

## 3. How long has TIR been in use?

TIR has been in use since 1984 in something similar to its current form. It has undergone minor modifications over the years, mostly in the interests of greater simplicity and teachability.

## 4. What is the anticipated outcome of TIR?

In the great majority of cases, TIR correctly applied results in the complete and permanent elimination of most PTSD symptomatology. It also provides valuable insights, which the viewer arrives at quite spontaneously, without any prompting from the facilitator and hence can "own" entirely as his own.

By providing a means for completely confronting a painful incident, TIR can and does deliver the mastery of the situation a person would have had if he had been able to fully confront the trauma at the time it occurred.

## 5. What are the contraindications and risks of TIR?

TIR is contraindicated for use with clients who:

a. Are psychotic or nearly so. TIR is most definitely an exposure or uncovering technique and hence is not appropriate for such clients.

b. Are *currently* abusing drugs or alcohol. Clients should avoid taking painkillers, sleeping pills, tranquilizers or drugs which may impair their physical or mental abilities for at least 24 hours prior to a viewing session. Some substances require a longer abstinence before viewing can take place.

c. Are not making a self-determined choice to do TIR. For TIR to work, the client has to want to do it. If the client is there under duress (e.g., on court order) or trying to please someone, TIR will not work. It may be possible, however, to explain to a reluctant client what TIR is. The client must be motivated to do the work before starting.

      d. Are in life situations that are too painful or threatening to permit them to concentrate on anything else. If the client is afraid of being murdered or engaged in violent fighting with his spouse, for instance, such issues/situations would have to be addressed first by consultation to develop a plan to handle the current life situation before the client will be ready to do TIR.

      e. Have no interest in or attention on past traumas. A general rule is to follow the interest of the client. The larger subject of Applied Metapsychology includes a large array of techniques that help a viewer to bring greater order and certainty to her mental environment.

Since the TIR technique is completely client-centered and non-forceful, clients will protect themselves if they are getting in too deeply by simply discontinuing the procedure. Hence there are no negative effects from properly facilitated TIR. If the facilitator were to try to force the client to run an incident, TIR could cause a considerable (though temporary) upset. But one of the cardinal Rules of Facilitation (see http://www.tir.org/metapsy/rules.htm) is never to force the client and always to follow the client's interest. Since we follow the client's interest at all times, we don't encounter resistance. If the client resists, we consider that we are not addressing the material the client should be looking at, at present.

## 6. What are the historical antecedents of TIR?

TIR grew mainly out of the work of Carl Rogers and Sigmund Freud. In *Two Short Accounts of Psycho-Analysis*, Freud describes a method to resolve sequences of similar traumas:

      What left the symptom behind was not always a *single* experience. On the contrary, the result was usually brought about by the convergence of several traumas, and often by the repetition of a great number of similar ones. Thus it was necessary to reproduce the whole chain of pathogenic memories in chronological order, or rather in reversed order, the latest ones first and the earliest ones last; and it was quite impossible to jump over the later traumas in order to get back more quickly to the first, which was often the most potent one.

Freud later abandoned this technique in favor of free-association. It seems likely that (in retrospect) the reason it didn't work well was the degree of interference the analyst introduced by interpretations and by forcing the analysand [client] in various ways, and the lack of a systematic, repetitive approach to achieving the desired anamnesis.

The work of Carl Rogers was invaluable in providing rules – such as a proscription against interpretations and evaluations – and an overall viewpoint of respect for the authority of the client, both of which we use to help create a safe environment for running TIR.

Although Rogers first described his work as "non-directive" and later as "person-centered", it seems obvious that "non-directive" doesn't mean the same thing as "person-centered". "Person-centered" describes the attitude of respect for the superior authority of the client and the concomitant rules for not stepping on the client's reality. "Non-directive" means the client gives structure to the session. These two are actually separate dimensions (see Fig. 1). For instance, classical, free-associative psychoanalysis is non-directive, but not person-centered. Cognitive and behavioral therapies are non-person-centered (because the therapist disputes the reality of the client) and directive (the therapist determines the agenda). Rogers is non-directive and person-centered. TIR falls into the fourth category: person-centered and directive, as the TIR facilitator provides structure for the client to be able to do the work of the session.

| *Directive* | **Cognitive and Behavioral Therapies** | **TIR and Applied Metapsychology** |
|---|---|---|
| *Non-Directive* | **Classical, free-associative psychoanalysis** | **Pure Rogerian** |
| | ***Non-person centered*** | ***Person-centered*** |

Dimensions of Direction and Person-Centeredness (Fig. 1)

# 7. How and why does TIR work?

Freud based his work on the theory that in order to recover from past traumas, it is necessary to achieve a full anamnesis (recovery of lost memory). He never adequately explained *why* anamnesis was necessary; however let's consider a person centered explanation.

A trauma, by definition, is an incident that is so painful, emotionally or physically, that one tends to flinch away from it, not to let oneself be aware of it, or, in Freud's terms, to repress it. It is the *flinch* and not the objective content of the incident that makes it a trauma. An event that is challenging and exciting for one individual may be traumatic for another. The one for whom it is a mere challenge is able to "stay with it" and master it; the one who experiences it as a trauma is usually not.

By definition, then, a trauma contains repressed material. Contained in a trauma, too, is one or more intentions. At the very least, there is the intention to push it away, to blot it out, to repress it. And there are usually other intentions as well, such as the intention to fight back, to get revenge, to run away, or (quite commonly) the intention to make sure that nothing like this incident ever happens again.

> *By definition, then, a trauma contains repressed material.*

An activity continues so long, and only so long, as the corresponding intention exists. That means that for each ongoing intention, there is an activity (at least a mental one) that continues as part of the here and now.

People subjectively define time in terms of the activity they are engaged in. Objectively, time is a featureless continuum. But subjectively, time is divided up into chunks—periods of time. For every given activity (and for every given intention) there is a corresponding period of time, and so long as you have an intention, you remain in the period of time defined by that intention (and activity). Holding onto an intention holds you in the period of time that commenced with the formulation of that intention. There are only two ways of ending an intention:

1. Fulfilling the intention, whereupon it ends spontaneously. You can't keep intending to win a race after you have won it.

2. Unmaking it. Even if you don't fulfill an intention, you can decide not to have that intention anymore and cause it to end. This, however, requires a conscious decision. You have to be aware of the intention and why you formed it.

But what if the intention is buried in the middle of a repressed trauma? In this case, neither condition (1) nor (2) can be satisfied, and the intention persists indefinitely. The person remains in the period of time defined by that intention, i.e., *the person remains in the traumatic incident*. The incident floats on as part of present time and is easily triggered (i.e., the person is easily reminded of it, consciously or unconsciously).

The only way a person can exit from that period of time (and from the intentions, feelings and behaviors engendered by the trauma) at which point the following becomes clear:

a. What intentions were formulated at the time of the incident.

b. Why they were formulated at that time.

Then, and only then, one can satisfy condition (2), above, for ending an intention, and one can let go of the intention. Without a thorough anamnesis, condition (2) cannot be satisfied.

## 8. How does TIR compare with other techniques for addressing traumatic stress?

*Please see Chapter 10 in Beyond Trauma: Conversations on Traumatic Incident Reduction, 2nd Ed. (2005)*

## 9. How can I find out more about TIR or find a practitioner?

Visit www.TIR.org

## 10. How can one get trained in TIR?

You can learn TIR by taking the basic TIR Workshop from a certified TIR trainer. Consult the Traumatic Incident Reduction Association website as above in order to find the nearest certified trainer.

## 11. What are the prerequisites for training?

A willingness and intention to help others and a reasonable degree of intelligence.

# Index

www.ingramcontent.com/pod-product-compliance
Lightning Source LLC
Chambersburg PA
CBHW080331270326
41927CB00014B/3176